Stretch to Win

Ann Frederick
Chris Frederick

HUMAN
KINETICS

Library of Congress Cataloging-in-Publication Data

Frederick, Ann, 1961-
   Stretch to win / Ann Frederick, Chris Frederick.
      p. cm.
   Includes bibliographical references and index.
   ISBN-13: 978-0-7360-5529-1 (soft cover)
   ISBN-10: 0-7360-5529-0 (soft cover)
   1. Stretching exercises.   I. Frederick, Chris.   II. Title.
   RA781.63.F74 2006
   613.7'1--dc22

                                            2006003700

ISBN-10: 0-7360-5529-0
ISBN-13: 978-0-7360-5529-1

The Web addresses cited in this text were current as of April 2006, unless otherwise noted.

Acquisitions Editor: Ed McNeely; **Developmental Editor:** Julie Rhoda; **Assistant Editor:** Carla Zych; **Copyeditor:** Elizabeth Foz; **Proofreader:** Kathy Bennett; **Indexer:** Nan N. Badgett; **Permission Manager:** Carly Breeding; **Graphic Designer:** Nancy Rasmus; **Graphic Artist:** Sandra Meier; **Photo Manager and Photographer (interior, unless otherwise noted):** Dan Wendt; **Cover Designer:** Keith Blomberg; **Photographer (cover):** Dan Wendt; **Art Manager:** Kareema McLendon-Foster; **Illustrator:** Argosy; **Printer:** United Graphics

Human Kinetics books are available at special discounts for bulk purchase. Special editions or book excerpts can also be created to specification. For details, contact the Special Sales Manager at Human Kinetics.

Printed in the United States of America   20   19   18   17   16   15

The paper in this book is certified under a sustainable forestry program.

Human Kinetics
Web site: www.HumanKinetics.com

United States: Human Kinetics
P.O. Box 5076
Champaign, IL 61825-5076
800-747-4457
e-mail: humank@hkusa.com

Canada: Human Kinetics
475 Devonshire Road, Unit 100
Windsor, ON N8Y 2L5
800-465-7301 (in Canada only)
e-mail: info@hkcanada.com

Europe: Human Kinetics
107 Bradford Road
Stanningley
Leeds LS28 6AT, United Kingdom
+44 (0)113 255 5665
e-mail: hk@hkeurope.com

Australia: Human Kinetics
57A Price Avenue
Lower Mitcham, South Australia 5062
08 8372 0999
e-mail: info@hkaustralia.com

New Zealand: Human Kinetics
P.O. Box 80
Torrens Park, South Australia 5062
0800 222 062
e-mail: info@hknewzealand.com

We dedicate this book to all of our athletes—the professionals as well as all the others who are committed to excellence in athletic performance—as without them it simply would not have been possible. Words cannot adequately express our deep gratitude and appreciation for the confidence and faith that they have placed in our work. It was only through a mutual willingness to build and maintain deep, honest, and trusting relationships that we were able to help them meet and surpass their goals of optimal performance and injury prevention. We celebrate the success that they have achieved with us by sharing the knowledge that we have gained.

contents

acknowledgments

The journey that has led to the development of our technique has been in progress for over 40 years and will continue for as long as we practice, so there are many people to thank.

This book would not have been possible without my beloved husband, Chris. He was instrumental in the entire creative process and has been my true partner. We spent countless hours working together on the book, side by side on our dueling laptops, without a single disagreement. Although I had spent many years studying the science of flexibility and stretching people before we met in 1997, his inspiration, guidance, support, vision, and love transformed my work and helped it evolve.

I especially want to thank my parents for having always been there for me, believing in and supporting all my dreams and endeavors. They generously opened their home to me as I completed my college degree and got the company up and running. My mom taught me that I could become anything I desired as long as I kept my feet planted firmly on the earth and my spirit reaching for the heavens. My father advised me to find a special niche, become the very best at it, and never stop improving.

Numerous influences have culminated in the present beliefs Chris and I share about stretching and flexibility as a means of tapping into human potential, beginning with our mutual backgrounds in dance and movement. I began dance training at the age of 4, and Chris began dancing at the age of 10. Thanks to the multitude of dance teachers and students I have had the pleasure of working with over the past 30 years for providing endless inspiration as to all the possibilities that exist in movement and flexibility.

Special thanks to Tim McClellan and Rich Wenner, who introduced me to the world of strength and conditioning at Arizona State University in 1995. They gave me a chance to develop my techniques into a functional flexibility that transferred to the field for athletes. This opened the door to my being chosen as the flexibility specialist for the 1996 U.S. Olympic Wrestling team. The experience of working with athletes of this caliber set the benchmark for the role sport-specific flexibility can have in athletic success.

Thanks to Beverly Kearney, head coach for the ladies track team at the University of Texas, for allowing us into the incredible world of human speed and perseverance inhabited by Beverly, her staff, and her amazing athletes. It was a gift to be a part of this world and to share in the glory and grit of competition for the Texas Relays and the preparation for the 2000 and 2004 Olympics.

I must thank my many clients over the past 12 years for believing and trusting in me and my work. By sharing their lives and providing feedback, they have participated in the development and growth of my vision. They have taught me a great deal about the many differences and similarities in the human body and about its unlimited potential.

A very special thank-you to my athletes for the time, trust, and devotion they have invested in me over the years. They have truly inspired me to continue improving the methods of stretching in order to help them reach their performance, injury prevention, and health goals. It has been an honor and a privilege to be a small part of their careers. We are especially grateful to the dozen NFL clients who took time out of their demanding schedules to act as models for the book: Steve Bush, Chris Cooper, Russell Davis, Na'il Diggs, Donovan McNabb, Casey Moore, Scott Peters, Scott Player, Neil Rackers, Josh Scobey, L.J. Shelton, and Fred Wakefield.

A simple thank-you is not sufficient for one very important athlete and client of ours, Donovan McNabb, who exemplifies the best of what an athlete, leader, and man can be. We have been fortunate to share in his exciting and eventful professional NFL career. His strong conviction that flexibility is the crucial factor in long-term athletic success and his support of our technique have been of great benefit to us, professionally and personally. He truly embodies the power of flexibility and is our Stretch to Win poster man!

Ann Frederick

First and foremost, I would like to thank my wife. This book is a product of and a testament to the joy that comes when we have the opportunity to create something together. I will never forget the first time I got on Ann's table and through her stretching techniques experienced the magical sensation of pain and tension melting away, the feeling shared by all her clients every day. She is a master teacher and a divine inspiration, and I thank her for personally training me in her original philosophy and system of stretching and for sharing with me all the things that drive her passion in this field.

Thanks to my parents for encouraging me to follow my heart in all my endeavors, even when the path I chose was not exactly what they had in mind for me. A very special thank-you to the first teacher and person who made a significant impact in my life, Sifu Sat Chuen Hon, for helping me create a solid spiritual and physical foundation. Special thanks to Dr. Mei-Hsiu Chan, for her current guidance in reaching deeper levels of life experience through profound training of the body and mind.

Thanks to all the dance teachers who freely gave of themselves when teaching their passion and joy of movement to me: Wilhelm Burrman, David Howard, Melissa Haydn, Gloria Fokine, and the late Robert Blankshine.

I thank my mentor and guide in manual therapy, Marika Molnar, PT, LAc. Without her inspiration, I would not be the kind of manual physical therapist that I am proud to be today. Liz Henry, PT, and Katie Keller, PT, were also wonderful guides on that journey.

There are many others who contributed to the creation of this book. A very special thanks to Michael J. Alter, whose first book in 1988, *The Science of Stretching*, provided scientific validation of an emerging field called flexibility science. Michael laid the groundwork and inspiration for others to follow, and we hope that we do his work some justice. He was kind enough to share his valuable time and knowledge in reviewing our manuscript, sending research, and discussing the future of flexibility science. Thanks also to Wayne Phillips, PhD, our dear friend and colleague, who was instrumental in the pursuit of research in the field, and to Jim Oschman, PhD, who was inspirational in his brilliant work relating to the wonders of the fascial system. Special thanks to Tom Myers, who gave us a brand-new perspective on how to see and experience the body. After spending 12 weeks training with him in Maine, being exposed to the tremendous volume of work covered in his book *Anatomy Trains*, we can truly say that we "changed our body about our mind." Cheryl Soleway's introduction of the FitBALL for self-myofascial release had a big impact on our thinking and practice. A special thank-you to Benny Vaughn, one of our most valued colleagues, who taught us a great deal through his vast experience, insight, and clarity as a fellow practitioner and one of our best students. His invaluable guidance, friendship, and support of our institute have shown us the meaning of great teaching.

Thanks to all the students who have trained in our technique, for their trust, time, passion, and commitment. They motivate us to be our very best and to continue evolving. We learn so much from them every time we teach, and we are eternally grateful for their constant faith and never-ending inspiration. Thanks also to our models—Lewis Elliot, Sonia Kang, and Liz Sambach—for donating their time and talent.

Extra thanks to Barbara Davis, our office manager extraordinaire. She has been fantastic in putting up with the lunacy for the past three years that this book has been in progress and the impact it has had on our office.

Last but certainly not least, we would like to thank the fine folks at Human Kinetics who have literally made this book possible: Ed McNeely, who took me seriously when I asked him, "When are you guys going to write a book for functional flexibility that the athletes can really use?" and called six months later to ask, "How would you like to write that book?"; Ted Miller, who understood our crazy schedule demands and adjusted deadlines in order to accommodate us and allow us to focus on our practice; and Julie Rhoda, our developmental editor, who was a pleasure to work with and was extremely helpful and understanding throughout the entire writing process. Thanks also to the HK editorial staff and freelancers for their help in refining our work to achieve greater clarity in presenting our system. We thank photographer Dan Wendt for his beautiful work, and the artists for doing a marvelous job interpreting and illustrating our ideas. Finally, we thank all those we don't know by name who had a part in helping this book come to fruition.

Chris Frederick

introduction

Whether they are training for football, golf, a 10K running race, or any sport in the Olympics, most athletes recognize the performance benefits of a progressive strength and conditioning program. However, stretching programs are often less popular, for a variety of reasons. Research on stretching has produced mixed reviews. The physical changes resulting from a stretching program may not be as outwardly apparent as the muscle-mass development that takes place in just eight weeks of strength training in a healthy adult. Therefore, stretching is not perceived as the most productive use of time for an athlete, as is evident in many training programs designed for high-school, college, and even professional athletes.

When athletes stretch at all, they usually do so ineffectively, performing the same old-school stretching exercises that several generations of athletes and coaches have used. These programs often consist of holding the familiar positions to stretch the groin, hamstrings, hip flexors, and low back at the same intensity and for the same duration, day in and day out, regardless of the sport or the particular activities that the athlete will be engaging in that day. Or, even worse, a program may entail many repetitions of quick, jerky stretches (often with the aid of a band or rope) that are supposed to warm up the muscles right before practice or competition. In both cases, the athletes are likely to be worse off than they would have been if they hadn't stretched at all.

So, is a stretching program just as important as a strength and conditioning program for optimal athletic performance? Yes—if the stretches are performed correctly. This is not just a matter of finding an accurate position to stretch in; it's also a matter of using appropriate training parameters to get the most benefit from the stretch. It means properly warming up the body and developing each specific type of stretch and its intensity, duration, and frequency.

Of course, you cannot establish these parameters unless you first evaluate your flexibility, or range of motion (ROM). Once the results from the evaluation are in, you can design an individualized program to increase your sport-specific flexibility. Instead of a generic stretching program, you can have a refined flexibility training program that will be much more responsive to your individual needs as they change over time. The comprehensive evaluation will also help you establish a baseline of flexibility that you can refer back to periodically when you reevaluate your progress. This way, you are sure to meet your ROM and sport performance goals. The program of stretching may be set up in special intervals or periodized over the course of a year to complement your other sport training.

In this book, we start by explaining the how, why, where, and when of stretching so that you have a good reason to try the Stretch to Win system of flexibility training. Once you have this base knowledge, we present the easy-to-follow programs that will immediately start to make a major difference in your sports performance. If the thousands of clients we have worked with are any indication of the benefits of our system, you will experience more power, more strength, more endurance, and more flexibility than you have ever experienced up to now. What's more, you will eliminate or greatly reduce the incidence and prevalence of injuries and of all types of pain. One of our clients, Brian Dawkins, Pro Bowler safety of the Philadelphia Eagles, notes, "My coaches and team mates asked me what I was doing different because I was moving so much better on the field. I told them that I was doing the Stretch to Win program and it was getting me right."

Professional and elite athletes come to use this system because we provide a complete and clinically proven way to develop sport-specific flexibility. Ever since Ann Frederick showed in her master's-level thesis in 1997 that this system resulted in greater (36 to 52 percent) and longer-lasting gains in range of motion than conventional methods of stretching, we have been constantly refining and improving the system. (In fact, now we get permanent ROM gains of between 50 and 125 percent in our clinic.) This guarantees that our clients, our students, and you are getting the most up-to-date and cutting-edge information and techniques to optimize athletic performance and to reduce the time it takes to return to activity after injury or surgery.

The Stretch to Win system aligns with today's philosophy of functional outcome training. This means that when you implement the program you are not just stretching to increase ROM for the sake of improving general mobility, but rather you are performing a specific stretch program based on an analysis of your own flexibility requirements specific to your sport or movement. In our experience, customized programs always lead to superior results.

A stretching exercise is functional when it directly enhances an athlete's performance in his or her specific sport. For example, a 100-meter sprinter should stretch differently than a marathoner. This is because the sprinter has faster-responding muscles owing to her higher percentage of fast-twitch fibers.These fast-twitch fibers help produce explosive power from start to finish in a sprint. The marathoner tends to have a higher percentage of slow-twitch muscle fibers than the sprinter. These slow-twitch fibers are accustomed to a much longer duration of performance, and hence do more to maintain correct postural alignment and form during distance running.

Another difference between these two athletes is the contrast between their ROM requirements. The sprinter must start a race crouched down in the starting blocks, while the marathoner begins positioned upright in ready stance at the starting line. In addition to being fast, the sprinter must have sufficient flexibility to start off the blocks effectively. When an athlete stretches using a training system that incorporates principles of sport-specificity, he or she can achieve optimal functional flexibility.

The idea behind this book is to provide athletes and coaches with the tools to create an effective flexibility program that contributes to optimal performance in any sport or training activity. An equally important goal is to eliminate the myths and confusion surrounding the subject of stretching and flexibility training and to educate and inspire readers with all of the new information and training that we have been fortunate enough to be immersed in as specialists in human flexibility. Before we help you create the program, we teach you how to evaluate your mobility and identify your restrictions to unhindered athletic movement. After you come up with objective findings about what imbalances and flexibility deficiencies you have, you will learn how to individualize your program to fit your needs. When you finally engage in a program that is suited to your particular needs, you will experience what our professional athlete clients get from us—faster and greater gains in ROM. These results will be evident after the very first time you perform the program, and they'll get cumulatively better over the following two weeks.

Chapter 1 takes you through the 10 basic principles of our program, the fundamentals for mastering the system. As you know from participating in sports, you must master the fundamentals before progressing to the next level. In chapter 2, we help you understand athletic flexibility: where it comes from, how and why you get tight, and what you can do to get more flexible. You will get to know all the possible factors that can affect your flexibility. For example, our clients who play in contact sports have noticed an enormous difference in how well they feel when they wake up in the morning and how well they perform if they've done a brief customized stretching routine within an hour of falling asleep the night before. With this knowledge, they are able to stretch more effectively and make the results last longer.

In chapter 3 we relate flexibility to performance and help you identify key indicators that point to problems in functional range of motion that you probably never gave much thought to before. These are the things that plague many athletes' performances throughout their careers if never identified and corrected. We then discuss how the flow of an optimal flexibility program will determine the flow of athletic performance.

Chapter 4 helps you apply the information in the previous chapters by teaching you how to assess your own flexibility using a personal flexibility assessment (PFA)—an honest look at what may be holding you back in your athletic performance. Based on the findings in the PFA, chapter 5 then guides you in building a customized stretching routine around your particular needs, rather than stretching for its own sake.

Chapter 6 teaches you how to fit a flexibility program into any training you are already involved in for a seamless integration of total training. This is accomplished by working in what we call the *stretching matrix*, a system of stretches that starts with the core group of muscles and fascia that are most important for athletes and extends outward to other relevant muscle groups, based on your own flexibility and sport-specific needs. We teach you programs that take as little as 60 seconds or as long as 60 minutes, depending on your needs, your goals, and the time you have available. These programs can be done anywhere, using tools and support like balls, walls, and bands. We also discuss stretching in the steam room, sauna, and whirlpool.

In chapter 7, we detail illustrated sport-specific stretches and provide testimonies from professional athletes who have used the same stretches. You will learn how to create safe, individualized stretches that are effective for bringing your body back to balance after hard training or athletic competition. Finally, in chapter 8 we give you an idea of what we do with assisted stretching to help our elite and professional athletes reach optimal levels of performance. This final chapter is intended for the professional who has a background and experience in anatomy, kinesiology, and manual therapy. The chapter will also be helpful for those of you who are not so trained but who want to find someone to assist you in stretching.

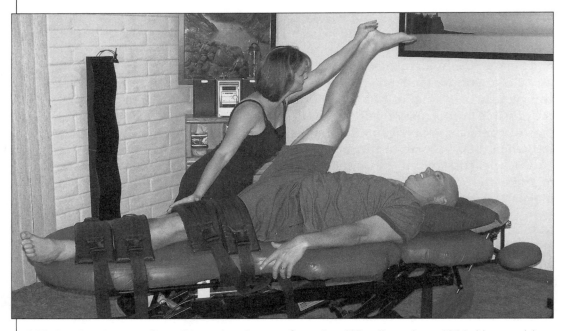

NFL Pro Bowl punter Scott Player has been a Stretch to Win client since 1999. He considers stretching the most important aspect of his training and credits it with keeping him injury free. Player states, "It has allowed me to train year round and stay on top of my game."

This book reflects our passion for stretching and flexibility training. By taking advantage of the knowledge we've developed over years of work with our clients, you will gain much more than flexibility. You will save time by being more efficient in your training; you will save money by not having to depend so much on professionals to get you out of pain; you will achieve athletic goals that were previously out of reach; and you will enjoy training and sport participation more as you increasingly experience the natural high of being in the moment where everything fits into the right place at the right time. For the ultimate athletic experience, you gotta stretch to win!

chapter 1

Ten Principles for Stretching Success

The goal of this book is to provide for athletes and for those who train them a method of stretching that is as effective and efficient as possible and that serves to enhance each athlete's performance, improve recovery after intense activity, and reduce the risk of injury. After a combined 40-plus years of experience, research, study, and professional practice as master instructors and coaches, we have identified 10 elements that form the foundation of the Stretch to Win system:

1. Synchronize your breathing with your movement.
2. Tune your nervous system to current conditions.
3. Follow a logical anatomical order.
4. Make gains in your range of motion without pain.
5. Stretch the fascia, not just the muscle.
6. Use multiple planes of movement.
7. Target the entire joint.
8. Use traction for maximal lengthening.
9. Facilitate body reflexes for optimal results.
10. Adjust your stretching to your present goals.

These 10 principles form the core of our system, yet like systems of the human body, they operate together in a nonlinear way. Therefore, the principles are not numbered in order of their importance, nor are they to be followed in strict order. Instead, they are organized to follow a multilayered, anatomical approach to function—from the deepest and simplest layer of movement that we started with in this world, breathing, to the outer reaches of highly complex, multiple planes of movement used in sports—to help you achieve your performance goals. The literal layers of anatomical sructure are located in regions of the body—joint capsules and fascia—that have traditionally not been fully addressed in other stretching and flexibility training programs. We have seen our clients change their flexibility and sport performance radically by following these principles, and you can experience the same success.

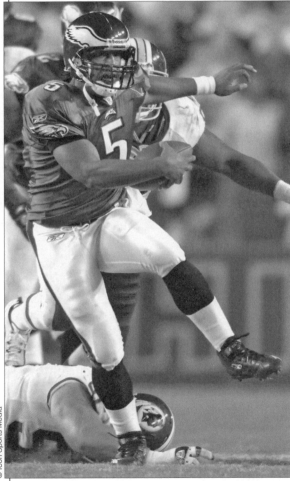

© Icon Sports Media

Donovan McNabb has been a client for many years and credits the Stretch to Win system for much of his success.

Principle 1: Synchronize Breathing and Movement

Donovan McNabb, NFL quarterback, has been using our system for the past seven years and is a great example of an athlete who understands the important role of breathing in influencing his mental, emotional, and physical state. Anyone who has tried to hit a target by throwing a ball, using a bow and arrow, or shooting a gun knows that the timing of breathing is crucial to hitting the target accurately.

The mechanical action of inhaling and exhaling works synchronously with your nervous system, which in turn influences your heart rate and blood pressure. Consequently, the way you breathe—the rate and rhythm—either revs up your system or calms it down. For example, if you voluntarily start to take rapid, shallow breaths, you have to increase the muscular effort in order to increase the rate of breathing. Increased muscular activity and rapid breathing are two states that cause a person to rely on secondary muscles of breathing (muscles other than the diaphragm, such as the muscles of the neck and rib cage). Both states occur because of increased impulses in the sympathetic nerves. This means that when bundles of nerves called sympathetic ganglia are stimulated (for example, when your rate of breathing increases), a flow of responses occurs to keep the body in a state of high alert. We discuss more details about the sympathetic nervous system (SNS) in chapter 2 (page 30).

We have discovered over the years that instead of counting how long to hold a stretch, athletes can stretch better by synchronizing their breathing with their movement. Counting puts an arbitrary time constraint on the stretch that competes with the actual release of the restricted tissues. Our experience has shown repeatedly that if the athletes instead focus on how they are breathing during a stretch, they get an optimal response from the stretch as well as an increased awareness of their bodies. They realize that their muscles and tissues have their own biological time clock for responding to a stretch that does not follow some prescribed formula or arbitrary time limit. Rather, it follows the state of the tissues and what they require at that moment. In this way, the breath actually assists the stretching movements by easing rather than forcing the athlete into increasing ranges of motion. By focusing on breathing, an athlete is also better able to gauge and adjust how much mental or physical tension he or she brings to the stretch.

> Breathing sets up your rhythm, whether you're training or in a game.
>
> *Donovan McNabb, 2005 Super Bowl quarterback, Philadelphia Eagles*

In many sports, if you breathe rapidly when you are supposed to relax, as when you are putting in golf, it makes focusing, concentrating, and being in the moment difficult, if not impossible. By contrast, if you tried to breathe very slowly when running or swimming a 100-meter sprint, then you really are not synchronizing your activity with your breathing. In either case, an inappropriate breathing technique negatively affects performance.

To see how this connection between breathing and performance works at a basic level, try this simple exercise:

1. Stand with your feet parallel to one another and placed directly beneath your hips.

2. Center your weight on the arches of your feet such that your weight is not concentrated on either your heels or your toes.

3. Slightly bend your knees without generating tension in your thighs.

4. Imagine your tailbone dropping to the floor and your head floating up to the ceiling, like a helium balloon.

5. Close your eyes and focus on your abdomen as it slowly relaxes and expands with each inhalation and relaxes and contracts with each exhalation.

6. Notice any areas of tension, discomfort, or pain; then return to the same breathing noted previously, feeling yourself breathing more fully and becoming more relaxed with each breath.

7. Remain in this state for a count of 10, one count being a full, slow inhalation and exhalation.

When our clients perform this basic awareness exercise, we hear a range of responses, including "I never knew how much tension I carry in my body" and "I never realized how hard it is for me to relax; why can't I relax?" We have also heard responses like "The pain that I had in my shoulder before this exercise is now gone!" What our clients have learned from this simple exercise is that they can become much more aware of regions in the body where they store unnecessary tension. More important, through specific instruction they learn how they can release any tension spontaneously and immediately through breathing. By contrast, if you perform the exercise again, this time with rapid chest breathing rather than slow breathing from the abdomen, you will note just how much tension you can generate after achieving the previous state of relaxation. The slow-breathing exercise is especially good for highlighting the relationship between tension and relaxation. After you perform this exercise the linear connection between breathing and the state of your body becomes obvious, providing a launching pad from which you can use this awareness in more advanced and specific ways.

We have observed in ourselves and in our clients that if you take this experience and knowledge of how breathing can influence muscle tension and apply it to stretching, the response you get from stretching is far better than it would be if you did not use this skill. This is because you learn how to accurately assess the current state of your body—relaxed or tense—through synchronized breathing (and the other nine principles) and give it what it needs at that moment. This may mean something as simple as recognizing unnecessary tension and releasing it in less time than it takes to take a complete breath, as you may have done in the previous exercise. Or it may mean taking a little time before going to sleep to go through a short stretching sequence that quickly restores your flexibility by unwinding and releasing the accumulated tension of the day. When our clients perform these recovery stretches and focus on their breathing instead of counting to an arbitrary number, they respond much quicker and with better flexibility. When you coordinate breathing and stretching in this way, you discover that certain areas of your body need less time and other areas need more time to release the restrictions to movement. When you learn to synchronize all your movements with proper breathing technique (as you will when we discuss the details in chapter 5), you will see profound changes in how you move on the athletic field or court, on the golf or ski course, and in activities of daily living.

Principle 2: Tune Your Nervous System

Tuning your nervous system enhances your flexibility for optimal athletic performance by preparing your body to meet the conditions at hand. The way you should stretch before a practice, training session, competition, or game (i.e., warming up) is very different from the way you should stretch after the activity (i.e., cooling down).

It is common knowledge in exercise science and sports medicine that a proper warm-up is essential for preparing the muscles and joints before engaging in full athletic activity, whether training or competing. To stretch or not to stretch as part of this warm-up has been a controversial question that has yielded research and anecdotal reports supporting both points of view. In practice, we find that it is not an all-or-nothing issue, but rather it is a relative issue of how and when to stretch appropriately for the given task.

In general, we have found that using the tenets of principle 1 and synchronizing your breathing with the type of stretching movement necessary for the intended result can attune your nervous system to respond to the conditions of the moment. If your intention is to warm up for a game or competition, then you want to tune your nervous system with a breathing and stretching movement style that increases blood flow to the muscles, increases focus and alertness in the mind and body, and generally prepares you to fully jump into the activity at the moment that you need to. Conventionally, stretching that includes these characteristics is called *dynamic stretching;* we instead use what we call *fast undulating stretching* (see chapter 5 for more details). Basically, in fast undulating stretching your breathing and stretching movements take on a quick pace characterized by a smooth flow of short-duration stretches with constantly changing positions of progressive amplitude so that oxygen and blood flow are maximally available to the mind and body for the athletic activities coming up. In scientific terms, this means that we need to create mental focus and stretch and adjust our breathing to prepare for activities that draw on the sympathetic nervous system.

In contrast, postactivity is a time for recovery and restoration of your flexibility, which might have suffered the effects of intense mental concentration and physical work. This is manifested by soreness and by what feel like ropes or knots in the muscles. Or, in the recent past you might have suffered a strain in the groin or hamstring that still makes you limp a little after you train or practice and is especially evident when your body has cooled down. In either case, whether a knot or a strain in the muscle, the goal is to restore the flexibility that was lost and to do it as quickly as possible so that you feel fresh and flexible in the morning and ready for activity again. Conventionally, static stretching has been prescribed for achieving these goals. Our system instead uses *slow undulating stretching.* In slow undulating stretching you want to tune the nervous system by synchronizing the breath and movement to a slower pace with progressively larger amplitudes of movement, moving through the positions for relatively longer durations than you held during the preactivity or fast undulationg movements. This results in stimulating the parasympathetic nervous system (PNS), which in simple terms decreases tension and muscle tone while relaxing the mind for a complete recovery from the day's activities.

Our clinical experience has shown us that when you tune the nervous system to the conditions you are preparing the body for, you enhance your ability to move as needed during the activity while reducing the risk of injury.

Principle 3:
Follow a Logical Anatomical Order

Our experience as dancers and martial artists and through stretching thousands of clients has shown that following the anatomical order of tissue layers when stretching produces the best results. In general, we have discovered that stretching the layers of the joint capsule, followed by the overlying deeper layers of muscles, before stretching the superficial layer results in better flexibility than when this order is not followed. The scientific reasons for this are complex and varied, involving multiple effects on the central and peripheral nervous systems. Suffice it to say that stimulating the relaxation and release of restrictions in the deeper structures of the body leads to a succession of reflexes and biochemical processes that paves the way for the rest of the body to respond to stretching in a much more profound way. We go into some detail on this in principle 7 (page 11) and in chapter 2 (page 28).

Clinically, we find tight, or hypomobile, hip joint capsules in a majority of our clients; this tends to be the first and deepest barrier of tightness that restricts flexibility and reduces efficiency of movement in the lower body. A common way to assess this is to lie on your back and pull one knee up to your chest, holding your knee with your hands. A pinching sensation in the hip or groin of the moving leg is a sign of hip impingement. This may be due to inflammation, but many more times it is simply from a tight hip joint capsule and hip flexors restricting movement. In fact, if you are very tight, you will probably also feel a stretch on the opposite hip, in the front or in the groin. Because the two opposing surfaces of the hip joint are abnormally compressed by the stiff joint capsule and tight muscles crossing the joint, it is possible that you will get arthritis in the hip if you continue to ignore this simple symptom. Fortunately, targeted stretching of this area can reduce the likelihood of developing this condition if you get to it in time.

After the joint capsule and shorter, single-joint muscles are made more flexible, the longer, multijoint muscles may be stretched more effectively as the layers of muscle and connective tissue, from deep to superficial and from short lengths to long lengths, are released in an easy-to-follow form.

Another logical sequence to consider is to prioritize stretching of the muscles that, because of severe tightness, inhibit proper functioning of muscles on the opposite side of a joint. A common example is a situation where tightness of the hip flexors inhibits proper contraction of the hip extensors. When hip extensors such as the gluteal muscles do not perform their actions appropriately, the hamstrings take on the extra workload. Since the hamstrings are synergists in helping the gluteals (or "glutes") to extend the hip, they become synergistically dominant in this scenario. Synergistically dominant muscles govern active movement when the prime movers (in this case the hip extensors) are not working. The all-too-common result in this scenario is that the hamstrings are strained or tear because of the extra workload they are not designed to accommodate. As soon as the excessive tension is removed through proper stretching (in this case, of the hip flexors), the muscles that were made weak by being inhibited (the hip extensors) immediately become strong and efficient and the strain in the synergists (the hamstrings) is eliminated.

Principle 4:
Gain Range of Motion Without Pain

Simply put, the philosophy of "no pain, no gain" is not part of the Stretch to Win system. Although it is traditional in some sports to take that approach toward increasing flexibility, we have found that we get better results by not eliciting the pain response.

In our clinic we have found that the most dramatic increases in flexibility and performance on the athletic field are created in an environment of quiet, relaxation, and trust. With these factors we have seen flexibility gains of between 50 and 100 percent with our tightest athletes by the first or second assisted stretch session. These gains were achieved without pain. With self-stretching, you can also achieve dramatic gain without pain after mastering these principles and applying them consistently in your program.

If an athlete has ever had the experience of feeling tighter or sorer after stretching, he or she probably stretched too intensively, was not breathing properly, or was not stretching appropriately for his or her goals. In fact, as testimony from some of our clients indicates, a number of athletes don't stretch because they feel they get tighter or sorer instead of looser after stretching. This result of stretching is unacceptable for competitive athletes. So how can they avoid this?

An important part of increasing ROM without pain is learning how to release or come out of a stretch while avoiding what we call the *rebound effect of stretching*. This effect refers to the tendency of muscle that has just been stretched to tighten up again either immediately or within a 48-hour delayed onset of muscle soreness, depending on the duration and intensity of the stretch. This may occur with a sudden or a more prolonged stretch to a muscle, as well as with a stretch of substantial intensity, resulting in microtears. A sudden or quick stretch elicits a sudden contraction or spasm, called a *stretch reflex* which is the body's effort to avoid further injury (Alter 2004). A stretch that is too deep or too prolonged also elicits a rebound tightening effect that is followed by soreness. When frustrated with results, some clients (especially martial artists) have told us that they have purposefully slipped into deeper, more intense stretches in an effort to make better gains in their flexibility, frequently with unfavorable results.

The rebound effect of stretching often occurs when people come out of a stretch in a manner that negates the stretch that was just performed. This leads to a less-than-optimal response to the stretch, and the results that come from such stretching—not much change in overall flexibility—don't seem to justify the time spent. Does this sound familiar to you? This is a very common complaint we get from new clients who have not had much success with stretching.

After performing a stretch, if you return to the starting position along the same path of movement in which you went down into the stretch, you will recontract the very muscle fibers that you were trying to release; this will counteract any of the gains you might have made with the stretch itself. Therefore, learning how to return to a neutral starting position without retensing the stretched muscles is another crucial key to optimal flexibility and increasing ROM without subsequent pain.

Principle 5: Stretch Fascia, Not Just Muscle

This is one of the most important principles to grasp, because the condition of the fascia—a specific type of connective tissue in your body—is just as important as the muscle, if not more so, in terms of gaining more usable flexibility. We discuss this in more detail in the next chapter, but generally, superficial fascia is a flexible connective tissue structure that attaches directly underneath your skin and covers your entire body. You may find it helpful to picture it as similar to a thick fishnet stocking through which nerves, blood vessels, fluids, and fat can all pass. There is another firmer and deeper layer of fascia—myofascia—that wraps itself in and around every muscle and continues to extend outward to attach to every tendon, ligament, and bone. Picture this layer as a tight-knit stocking that surrounds and invests muscles. Because myofascia connects muscle fiber to muscle fiber and larger muscle groups to other groups in distinct structural patterns and attachments, a person can never just stretch one isolated muscle. It's all connected!

Another way to think about myofascia is to use an image of human anatomical development that Thomas Myers, one of our teachers and the author of *Anatomy Trains*, taught us: "Think of the body as having been just one muscle that has subsequently subdivided into more than 600 fascial bags." Since each muscle is contained within a fascial bag that connects to other fascial bags that extend deeper into the muscle like a cobweb around each muscle fiber (more on this in chapter 2), stretching can affect far more than just one muscle. Therefore, instead of having our clients think about stretching individual muscles, we have had much more success having them think about stretching continuous lines of fascia, from short to long and from thin to thick. This mental image of stretching myofascia is far more anatomically accurate and effective than thinking about stretching individual muscles.

The professional football players we work with offer an excellent example of how stretching one muscle to relieve tightness or soreness does not work. These players commonly complain of chronically tight and sore hamstrings, despite doing daily hamstring stretches. Naturally, tight hamstrings negatively affect athletic performance and confidence. What we usually see in these players are extremely tight hip flexors and tight deep hip external rotators from repetitive exploding out of the football squatting stances. After we instruct them on how to release the tightness of the joint capsule along with the hip flexors and gluteal group, the tightness in the hamstrings is eliminated.

> If you're not stretching your fascia, you're not really stretching.
>
> *Brian Dawkins, 2005*
> *Super Bowl and*
> *Pro Bowl safety,*
> *Philadelphia Eagles*

The reason most stretching programs fail is that they do not address all the factors that limit ROM. The key to gaining optimal flexibility is understanding the three-dimensional structure and function of the body, specifically its myofascia. One example of applying this structural and functional understanding would be lining up multiple joints in the hip and leg along a certain angle before you rotate the leg to emphasize stretching a certain fascial connection. Another example would be learning how to thoroughly stretch your entire body along multiple planes of movement (discussed in the next principle). In exploring the three-dimensionality of how your body feels and responds under different conditions of stretching, you will get to know how, why, and where the fascia changes when it shortens, lengthens, tightens, or twists during athletic activity. This will help you understand the impact fascial change can have on your muscles and your athletic performance. Among the negative effects that can occur are muscle weakening, muscle fatigue, inefficient recruitment of muscle fibers, decreased motor coordination, and a host of other performance-reducing factors. Any of these things may occur because, as we have said previously, the condition of the fascia determines the condition of the muscle. Fortunately, if these effects are due to imbalances in the fascial structure of the body, you can eliminate all of them with a proper flexibility program.

Principle 6:
Use Multiple Planes of Movement

Without a precise three-dimensional assessment of posture, gait, flexibility, strength, and other functional movements related to your activity or sport, you do not have most of the objective information you need to create an optimal stretching program to enhance your performance or rehabilitate an injury. Yet even without a professional evaluation, understanding movement from a three-dimensional perspective greatly adds to your ability to improve athleticism with much less chance of injury. You'll get these benefits when you stretch using multiple planes of movement and then integrate this knowledge and experience with specific training appropriate for your sport (covered in chapter 7).

We have seen many times that even professional athletes stretch indiscriminately and irregularly and thereby perpetuate existing muscle imbalances. When you stretch your arms or legs equally without specific regard to one being tighter than the other, you are stretching into the path of least resistance, which only increases your *relative* flexibility. Relative flexibility is the range of motion that comes naturally or most easily for an athlete who is training, competing, or stretching. For example, if an athlete has a tighter quadriceps on the right side and stretches both quadriceps at the same intensity, duration, and frequency, the right quadriceps will very likely remain tighter than the left. Since the left quadriceps has more flexibility than the right, it is more responsive to stretching and the stretching comes more easily. Consequently, the athlete's relative flexibility of both quadriceps increases because of stretching, but an imbalance between the two quadriceps will still exist, since the stretching parameters for the tighter leg were never adjusted to take its lesser ROM into account.

Frequently, the tighter side remains tight even when it is stretched more than the other, looser side. This happens because somewhere along one or more fascial connections to the tight arm or leg are contributing factors that perpetuate the flexibility imbalance, preventing you from getting the results you were expecting from your stretching. Tightness that does not respond to stretching should be evaluated by a professional.

A proper evaluation by an experienced professional can reveal the source of the imbalance; you may also find these imbalances by conducting your own assessment (see chapter 4) when you reflect on how you move in multiple planes during activities of daily living, fitness training, and sport competition. After performing this self-analysis, you can learn how stretching in multiple planes—adding different angles to take advantage of the unique mobility of certain joints—is directly related to how you move in sports. Then when you combine multiple angles with other techniques when you stretch—such as adding extra emphasis to the origin or insertion of the myofascia—you get the superior results that you expect from individualized attention. This kind of attention is simply giving your body what it needs at the time that it needs it, no more and no less than that. By regularly following these principles, you will learn how to listen to what your body needs at the moment that your body communicates it. In this way, small problems do not develop into larger ones, and you optimize your athletic performance.

In chapter 6 we address stretching along multiple angles and planes of movement, including components of rotation, diagonals, and traction. The more these components are used as building blocks in custom-designing a flexibility training program, the more successful it will be.

Principle 7: Target the Entire Joint

The joint capsule is made up of fascia that encapsulates our joints and fuses with the ligaments that connect the bones to each side of the joint. Thomas Myers has demonstrated by anatomical dissection that there are deep continuous paths of fascial tissue that connect the joint capsule to the ligament and bone, go on to the tendon and muscle, continue to the next tendon and bone, and from there go on to the ligament and capsule of the next joint. This repetition of fascial connections can span the entire length of the body so that tightness in the sole of your foot, for example, can catalyze various symptoms and pain anywhere through the fascial tracks of your back up to the base of your skull. Since the joint and its capsule are located in the deepest part of the fascial tracks just described, the condition of the joint capsule determines the condition of the fascial tracks that cross over and connect the joints.

Almost 50 percent of a healthy person's lack of ROM at the joint has been suggested in research to be due to the tightness of his or her joint capsules (Johns and Wright 1962). Therefore, it makes sense to keep this structure optimally mobile. When the capsule gets tight, it has a nasty tendency to become adhered, or "glued down," to the underlying bone. Unlike normal joint capsules, which permit a certain freedom of motion, tight capsules such as those found commonly in professional athletes restrict range of motion. When full range of motion in a joint is inhibited, then range of motion in the muscle is also restricted, because muscles attach to bones and bones connect to other bones by way of joints. If range of motion in the muscle is restricted, compensations for the restrictions develop automatically, because the body is neurologically programmed that way. Since we are speaking about movement, the body will develop areas of more mobility in some joints (called hypermobile joints) to compensate for the lack of mobility in other joints (called hypomobile joints) in order to continue to operate functionally. For example, when one of the four articulations of the shoulder is restricted, one or more of the other articulations will get increased mobility over time to compensate for the lack of the restricted one. The longer the restrictions are present, the more the body compensates for those limitations to movement. Over time, the accumulated compensations become areas of pain and dysfunctional movement, forcing the athlete to seek professional help.

A common example that we see in the clinic is hip joint capsules that seem, in the athlete's words, to literally get "jammed up" into the joint. This leads to a functional shortening of the length of the leg, because the jammed-up hip has less space available in the joint for mobility of the bones. This shortening effect may also occur on the affected side in the sacroiliac and lumbar facet joints as well. Since the bones of the hip socket are not moving through their full excursion, the deep hip flexor muscles of the psoas and its neighbor, the iliacus, get very tight and restricted in their motion. This negatively changes how the athlete runs, jumps, and performs other athletic moves. Over time, hip bursitis, tendinitis, or arthritis may develop, depending on the factors that are present. An athlete can completely avoid or eliminate these scenarios by addressing the flexibility of the entire hip joint capsule.

When you include the whole joint capsule in a flexibility program, you must understand the basic function of that joint. Taking the hip joint again as an example, you need to understand that it is a ball-and-socket type of joint. This means that it can move in an infinite number of directions. Using this knowledge when you stretch means targeting all the prime directions of stretching the hip so that maximal functional flexibility is achieved for the complex movement required in sports and athletics (see also chapters 4 and 5).

We also provide some guidelines in chapter 8 as to when stretching the joint capsule alone is indicated or contraindicated in assisted stretching, based on the whether the hip is hypo- or hypermobile.

Principle 8: Use Traction

When you stretch, you are simply trying to get tissue that has become tight—whether it be fascia, muscle, tendon, or ligament—to lengthen. It would seem logical that when things in your body get compressed and come together, like the hip joint we previously described, you would want to pull them apart, or traction them, to get more space between them again. When we say traction here, we mean first creating space in your joints before stretching, like lifting yourself up, feeling tall, before you stretch to reach down and touch your toes. In principle 3, we discussed the necessity of stretching in an order—starting with the joint capsule, proceeding to the shorter muscles that span one joint, then progressing to other muscles and fascia. And in principle 7, we mentioned the study (which matches our own experience) showing that almost 50 percent of tightness is within the joint capsule and its surrounding ligaments. Therefore, when we evaluate an athlete's hip joint and find the joint capsule is tight, or hypomobile, the first thing we do is remove this specific restriction with traction.

The ideal way to stretch the joint capsule is to apply manual longitudinal traction to the joint at the proper angle and at the correct intensity, duration, and frequency. In the case of the hip joint, this means that the practitioner who is stretching the athlete physically pulls the leg so that a gap or stretch is created in the hip joint capsule (see chapter 8). After the practitioner gets the joint capsule warmed up and responsive to stretching with circular movements and traction, the next focus is to apply traction to and stretch the muscles that cross over this joint. This is because these muscles are the closest and deepest layers that will react to positive or negative changes in the joint capsule—and they are innervated by the same nerves that control resting tissue tone or tension as well as the nerves that make the muscles, with their fascia, contract and relax in response to all movements. These muscles are shorter in length and anatomically and functionally closer to the joint capsule than the muscles that cross two or more joints; when released, therefore, they pave the way for the longer muscles to release faster and more efficiently. This is achieved by combining this principle of using traction with that of principle 6, "Use multiple planes of movement," to get maximal lengthening of any tissue that has become tight and has caused pain or otherwise negatively affected athletic performance. Even though we have just described manual traction with the assistance of someone else, traction may also be used with great success by yourself, without any special equipment, if used in combination with the other nine principles.

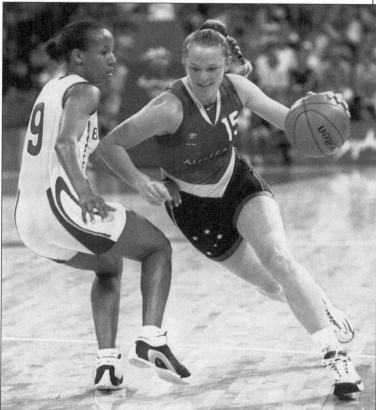

The ability to move well in multiple directions through all your joints depends on being flexible in all your tissue layers.

© Empics

When you get to stretching the muscles that cross multiple joints (called "multijoint" muscles), you add traction proximally and distally to get a complete myofascial stretch from the origin of the muscle to its insertion. In fact, the addition of traction in general amplifies the effects of stretching by going beyond mere local muscular attachments to related but distal fascial tracks, such as those mentioned in principle 7. These amplified effects include much greater ROM in the area being stretched as well as more permanent overall improvement in flexibility than stretching without traction brings.

In summary, the way to get maximal lengthening of tight tissue is to traction and stretch all the tissues along a fascial track—joint capsule, ligament, tendon, muscle—without pain. Move from the deep to the superficial layers, from myofascia that crosses one joint to that that crosses multiple joints, and then add multiple planes of movement as dictated by a synchronized breath and a properly tuned nervous system suited to the current conditions.

Principle 9: Facilitate Body Reflexes

Research in sport science and other disciplines repeatedly demonstrates that stretching using specific proprioceptive neuromuscular facilitation (PNF) techniques yields the most gains in range of motion in the shortest amount of time. PNF was developed in the 1940s as a complete system and philosophy of rehabilitation that used principles of neurological reflexes to improve the functioning of the body in people who had polio and other neurological disorders. Since research at that time demonstrated that PNF worked so well with that population, modified PNF techniques were developed for people who participated in athletics and wanted the benefits of increased flexibility and strength.

Recent research has demonstrated that the specific technique of modified PNF called contract-relax-agonist-contract (CRAC) and contract-relax (CR) has had the best overall results in improving flexibility. Our own research has shown that assisted PNF contract-relax stretching, combined with the use of special table straps to passively stabilize the nonstretched limb, results in even better and longer-lasting ROM (Frederick 1997). We describe our version of this technique, which we call undulating PNF, in chapter 8. Suffice it to say here that this technique employs well-known neurological reflexes that enable the body to take advantage of windows of opportunity in getting more range of motion and longer-lasting flexibility from stretching than would otherwise be possible.

Principle 10: Adjust Stretching to Your Goals

Three factors to consider when designing any training program are intensity, duration, and frequency of each component of the program. Determining the intensity of a stretch means knowing how far into the range of motion you can easily and safely go for the maximal effect. Duration refers to how long you hold the stretch to get the most gain in flexibility per stretch. Frequency means how often you must repeat the stretch sequences at one time or another over the course of the day to get optimal results specific to the task at hand.

To accomplish your individual goals for a stretching program, you will need to learn how to modify each of these three parameters to suit your needs. This is true for any effective program, and flexibility training is no exception. For example, if you feel tight on a given day, you will want to emphasize certain parameters, such as the frequency and duration of a stretch, more than others, such as the intensity. This is because you want to increase your flexibility without irritating or injuring your body, which can happen if you stretch too intensely. On the other hand, if you feel loose, then you will want to go through a brief but thorough flexibility program so that you can assess your body to make sure that all areas are indeed loose.

Not only will you learn how to adjust these parameters day to day, but these parameters can and should change over the course of your training depending on the season of training and the state your body and mind are in. These variables will affect how you design your flexibility program. Program design is covered in more detail in chapter 5.

Chapter 2 will help you understand the anatomy and physiology of flexibility and stretching. There, you will visualize the "blueprint," or layout, of the fascia of the body, which will lead to a better understanding of the hows, whats, and whys of stretching for better athletic performance.

Anatomy of Athletic Flexibility

When the Internet came into the mainstream it revolutionized the way people communicate with one another and operate their businesses. We increasingly depend on it because it is one of the most efficient ways to operate in today's world. The human body has existed for millennia functioning with similar communication systems of internets and intranets connected through a bodywide network. This physical network of your body is made up of a structural material called connective tissue. Since connective tissue is present everywhere in the body, as mentioned in principle 5 (pages 8 to 9), and since it has the ability to tighten or shorten as well as to stretch or lengthen, it makes sense to describe its structure so you can better understand its function in increasing flexibility.

Structure of Fascia

The basic unit of a human being is a cell; together cells form tissues such as organs, bones, muscles, and skin. As tissues of the same cells develop together, they form systems that function with other systems. It has become conventional to describe human anatomy and physiology in terms of the separate systems that operate together, and in the following section we follow this convention to some degree. An example is the skeletal system, which functions with the muscular and nervous systems, among others. Yet in truth there is only one integrated system of the human organism. Our aim is to show you how the function of this entire system is, to a great degree, dependent on the flexibility of the fascia.

As the human embryo develops, at a very early stage it differentiates into three distinct but interdependent kinds of cells—ectoderm, endoderm, and mesoderm layers. These three cell layers are the physical building blocks on which the entire structure of our body is made, forming the various tissues and organs. Connective tissue is formed from the mesodermal layer and, as the embryo develops, divides into four basic types: bone, cartilage, blood, and connective tissue proper. Connective tissue proper is further differentiated into dense, loose, reticular, and adipose tissues. Simply put, dense connective tissue forms ligaments and tendons, loose connective tissue holds organs in place, reticular connective tissue forms the soft part of our skeleton called the marrow, and adipose connective tissue's main role is to store energy in the form of fat, although it also cushions and insulates the body.

There is yet another specialized connective tissue layer called *fascia* which surrounds muscles, bones, and joints, providing support and protection and giving structure to the body. It consists of three layers: the *superficial fascia*, the *deep fascia*, and the *subserous fascia*. The superficial fascia is located directly under the first two layers of the skin, the epidermis and dermis. Its functions include the storage of fat and water, and it also provides passageways for nerves and blood vessels. In some areas of the body, such as the face, it also houses a layer of skeletal muscle, allowing for movement of the skin. The deep fascia is beneath the superficial fascia. It aids muscle movements and, like the superficial fascia, provides passageways for nerves and blood vessels. In some areas of the body, such as in the low back or lumbar and sacral region, it also provides an attachment site for muscles and acts as a cushioning layer between them. Subserous fascia is between the deep fascia and the membranes lining the cavities of the body. There is a potential space between it and the deep fascia which allows for flexibility and movement of the internal organs.

In order to keep a unified and simple approach when speaking about the connective tissues that can be influenced by stretching, we refer to them all as fascia, because all connective tissues are affected by stretching or lack thereof. When we want to speak about the fascia that specifically affects and influences muscles, we call it *myofascia*.

Before we go into the details of fascia, let's discuss what is common to all connective tissue so that you have the perspective of an integrated system rather than an isolated structure. Later in this chapter we discuss how this structural system functions beyond being a support for the body.

Extracellular Matrix

One of the defining features of connective tissue is that its cells are loosely positioned in an extensive matrix called ground substance (figure 2.1). Because this matrix occupies space outside the cell, it is called the extracellular matrix, or ECM. The ECM is produced by secretions from the cell and ranges in viscosity from free-flowing liquid (such as blood plasma) to a soft semisolid (such as the cartilage in the nose or ear) to solid substance (such as bone). As you can see in figure 2.1, blood vessels and nerves travel directly through the ECM. So when you stretch, it's good to keep in mind that these structures are stretching as well and may also be a source of tightness, pain, or even numbness. (Chapter 4 provides guidelines to help you avoid these symptoms while stretching.) In fact, nerves, arteries, and veins are made of specialized connective tissue, a fact that serves as more evidence that connective tissue structures are distributed throughout the body like a web or net.

The shape of the body's connective tissue may quickly and easily change in response to external or internal factors affecting the ECM. For example, you may have swelling and pain caused by fluid accumulating in the ECM or you may feel tight and sluggish when you are dehydrated because fluids leave the ECM. Such quick changes in the physical shape of your body are possible because of what connective tissue is primarily made of—collagen, elastin, and water. Collagen is the most abundant protein in humans and animals; as such it is also the most prevalent structural material in the human body after water. Its main structural property is its great tensile strength; therefore, tissues that contain more collagen than elastin, such as tendons, are resistant to pulling forces. Elastin, because of its unique biochemical and biophysical properties, is more elastic

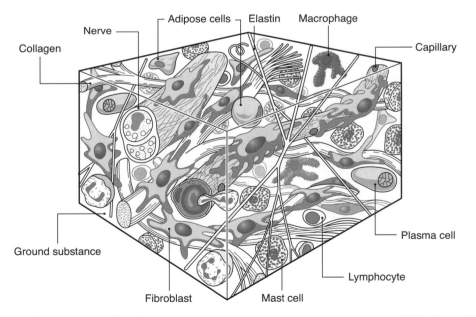

Figure 2.1 Connective tissue such as fascia is loosely positioned within the semi-viscous, gel-like exracellular matrix, or ECM.

than collagen. Therefore, tissues such as ligaments, which contain more elastin than collagen, allow more changes in their shape to occur. This is why athletes often avoid stretching ligaments in training—to keep them from becoming too loose and unstable. The third material, water, makes up about 60 percent of the body mass in males and 55 percent in females. According to Alter (2004), water makes up 60 to 70 percent of the total connective tissue mass in the body. Most of this water is in the blood and in the ground substance or ECM of connective tissue. Water has a physical property of high surface tension, which means that the surface layer behaves like a dynamic elastic sheet within blood vessels and connective tissue. This is part of the reason that, under nontraumatic conditions, soft tissue will yield without injury if you slip, fall, or collide with another athlete. Therefore, staying properly hydrated helps you prevent injuries.

In any case, the proportion of the amount of collagen to elastin to water in the ECM determines its structure and how the individual tissue functions. Because isolated collagen is resistant to tensile forces like stretching, tissues that have more collagen content will naturally be more resistant to stretching, even though elastin is present. Tissues with more elastin content will accept tensile forces and will tolerate stretching. This may explain why flexibility can vary a lot in an individual; one person's hips may be much tighter than the same person's shoulders because of a difference in the ratio between collagen and elastin. Unfortunately, elastic fibers have not been studied as extensively as collagen, but it has been established that collagen and elastin are very closely associated, as Alter (2004) put it, "anatomically, morphologically, biochemically, and physiologically." Therefore, even though you cannot know the exact proportion of elastin content around and in each and every muscle, tendon, and ligament, you can know how to take advantage of the properties of the fascia to keep it functionally optimal for assisting you in your activities.

One property of the ECM in the fascia that you can have some control in manipulating is the quality of viscoelasticity. Viscoelastic materials such as honey, Silly Putty, chewing gum, and polymer materials exhibit both the characteristics of a viscous liquid and an elastomeric solid. Viscoelastic materials behave more like solids at low temperatures and more like liquids at high temperatures.

The fascia behaves in the same manner. When you awaken, your body temperature is normally a degree or two lower than it is during the day; when you first move, you typically move slowly both because you are not quite clearheaded and because your body tissues are stiff. Your fascia is cooler and more viscous so it acts more like a solid (i.e., your body feels a lot slower and heavier) when you try to move quickly. Similarly, if you show up to train or compete in a sport, you know that you need to warm up the body first to prepare it to move at a faster pace requiring more strength, power, and agility.

After you have broken a light sweat is the time to take advantage of the heating and mobilizing effect on the fascia to stretch and prepare for the specific activity. In this case, you want to take advantage of the less viscous and more elastic properties of the tissue, so you will do faster-paced stretching to prepare for dynamic activity. After activity, the extracellular matrix is even less viscous and more like liquid, providing the perfect time to do slower-paced stretching that takes advantage of the fascia's plastic properties to restore and even increase length in the connective tissue, before it has a chance to cool down and get more solid again.

Unfortunately, it has been determined that with the aging process come changes to the connective tissue, among other things. As you age, collagen content increases in all tissues, and the quality of it decreases, resulting in increased stiffening of the body. Elastic fibers also lose their resiliency and undergo various changes including fragmentation, fraying, and calcification (Alter 2004). The fact that people tend to get more easily dehydrated as they age doesn't help matters, either. When we ask our veteran athlete clients about the one thing that has slowed their speed, agility, and quickness, they all reply that it is their loss of flexibility. Fortunately, it has also been determined that the more you stretch, the more your body produces the elements necessary to keep you flexible and to greatly diminish the stiffening effects of age (Oschman 2003).

Fascial Net

Since we live in a gravitational field, we are subject to forces acting to pull us downward toward the earth—unkind challenges to our balance and good looks! When the body does not have good structural alignment (i.e., good posture), it has to endure additional stress and strain in an effort to provide more support as it functions within the pull of gravity. You can think of the term stress as a structure under compression and the term strain as a structure under tension. Translated into symptoms, stress might feel as though something is being pressed on or squeezed, as when you sit for too long and your back feels like it is under pressure and needs to be stretched. Strain might feel like an uncomfortable pull in your back when you bend over, which makes you want to protect the area by staying well within your range of motion. Since we move in three dimensions with gravity, we always have both stress and strain at the same time. Figure 2.2, *a* and *b*, illustrates a good metaphor for the connective tissue in and around the spine and its viscoelastic properties.

On a basic level, similar kinds of forces make connective tissue do what the garden hose does in figure 2.2b. If you carry a heavy pail in one hand while walking, you tilt to the opposite side to accommodate the external force exerted on the body. If this is the case, then compression forces (or stress) that shorten tissue exist on one side while tensile forces (or strain) that lengthen tissue exist on the opposite side. If the viscoelasticity of the connective tissue is optimal, then when you release the heavy pail you return to your straightened posture with ease. If you have trouble straightening, your connective tissue system most likely has unbalanced regions. This could take the form of alternating zones of stress and strain in your body such that when additional forces like a heavy pail are exerted on it, it is incapable of appropriately handling the load. It may even reach a threshold level at which the connective tissue fails to adapt, resulting in

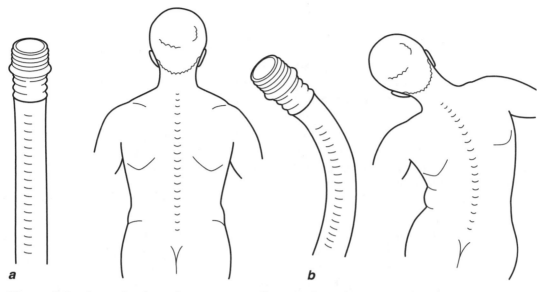

Figure 2.2 A garden hose is one way to illustrate how the connective tissue around the spine responds to simple forces (*a*). For example, if we bend the hose, (*b*) compressive forces generated from the action will deform the hose inward. In general, compression creates folds in semisolid, viscoelastic materials like our fascia. Figure *b* indicates tension being generated simultaneously on the concave side of the hose to make the hose bend or deform outward. In general, tension or tensile forces make materials fray, or split apart.

a sprained ligament or strained muscle. You can avoid these kinds of common injuries by keeping your connective tissue in optimal condition, as free as possible of accumulated stress and strain. The Stretch to Win system is one way to do that.

It is important to recognize that all these forces are constantly being exerted on you when you participate in sports or training and perform activities of daily living. In running, for example, the body must tolerate large ground reaction forces. This means that as hard and fast as you hit the ground, the ground sends the same force back through your body. Your ability as a runner to take those enormous forces and use them to assist you in running faster makes you a winner. When you are unable to handle those forces, structural imbalances in your body lead to injuries like stress fractures and tendinitis. This is why we teach you in chapter 4 how to evaluate your body's structural imbalances by analyzing your own posture and movement.

Part of what helps you handle these forces is the fabric of connective tissue, the fascia, that assists or resists your movements. The neuromusculoskeletal system is wrapped in this amazing material and depends on it to communicate information to and from the brain, spinal cord, and peripheral nerves. In fact, the brain and spinal cord are also wrapped in a special connective tissue called dura mater, and a whole discipline of manual bodywork called craniosacral therapy is based in part on the movement of fluids and the dura mater within this system.

So, in a sense, your brain is physically connected to the rest of you through this bodywide fabric, which for simplicity's sake we call the fascial network or fascial net. It is a network because it is part of the bodywide communication system that we cover in the next section. But it is also like a physical net in that it is a mesh of material made from threads—knotted, twisted, or woven to form a regular pattern with spaces between the threads. A net can also be visualized as a piece of mesh fabric in the form of a bag that is used for holding something. In sports such as soccer and hockey, nets are placed between goalposts to catch the fast-moving ball or puck. The trouble is, if a net—such as a basketball net—develops a kink or turns in on itself, then it does not serve its function and causes problems. The same trouble can happen in the fascial net.

We are mostly concerned with two layers of fascia: the superficial inner layer and the deep layer. The superficial inner layer allows the skin to slide and accept the types of forces that tend to shear the skin, such as when you roll over in bed or shift your position in a chair. We have also learned in our training as structural integrators that this layer tends to hold many of our superficial postural compensations, like bends, shifts, tilts, and rotations of the spine. The deeper layer (called the epimysium) lies in contact with the muscle and fuses with fascia that covers and connects tendons, bones, ligaments, nerves, and blood vessels. This is where the core of our postural imbalances, movement dysfunctions, and flexibility come from, especially around our low back, pelvis, and hips.

Even though tendons, ligaments, and bones have a different distribution of collagen, elastin, and water than the fascia that fuses with them, unless stated otherwise in this book we functionally group them all under the term *fascia*. This is because all of these tissues share the biomechanical effects of fascia; they all merge under the common influence of the fascial net. In fact, this net of fascia may also be thought of as an extensive cobweb that not only wraps around each muscle and around bundles of muscle fibers called fasciculi, but also differentiates and fuses with smaller and finer divisions of connective tissue, which in turn wrap around each muscle fiber all the way down to the molecular level of the single cell of a muscle, called a sarcomere (figure 2.3).

Therefore, how much and how long negative change has occurred in our connective tissue—from poor posture, too little movement, overtraining, injuries, and so on—will determine how many compensations are reflected in our fascia. When we were born, our fascia was clear and direct in its architecture, like clear plastic wrap defining the shapes and connections of our muscles, and with a perfect balance of collagen, elastin, and water. After years of negative changes, the fascia will twist, compress, and tighten in some areas while becoming overly lengthened and tense in other areas, negatively affecting the anatomy and physiology of our muscles as well as the rest of our body.

Another effective way to visualize the extent of fascia is to imagine a life-sized holographic computer model of a human from which you can delete all the skin, muscle, bone and fluids. You would still be able to see the full three-dimensional shape of the model, but its form would be defined instead by lines, sheets, and

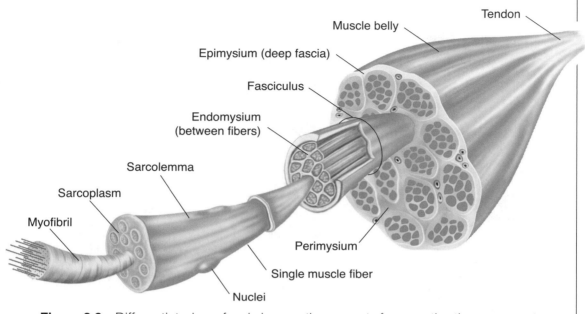

Figure 2.3   Differentiated myofascia is a continuous net of connective tissue present within and around the components that make up muscle, from the tendon and muscle belly all the way out to the sarcomeres within the myofibril.

Reprinted, by permission, from G.R. Hunter, 2000, Muscle physiology. In *Essentials of strength training and conditioning*, edited by T.R. Baechle and R.W. Earle (Champaign, IL: Human Kinetics), 4.

bags of fascia devoid of bone and muscle tissue. Unfortunately, since fascia as a system is still a relatively new concept, there has not been a human dissection or even a good drawing that shows it in its entirety. But if we had a complete computerized model depicting the full extent of our fascia, you would still see the entire nervous and circulatory systems, since both are formed by distinct specialized connective tissues. While we are most occupied here with the fascia of muscle, called myofascia, be aware that when we talk about flexibility we are talking about all of the connective tissue that makes up the fascial network, or simply, the fascial net. If muscles get tight, so do the nerves and blood vessels that supply them. When you stretch the fascial net, you need to know what you are stretching as well as how, why, and when to do it, since what you stretch and how you stretch it dictates the location and type of effect generated by the stretch.

Fortunately, Thomas Myers, a colleague and a teacher of structural integration, has created an effective diagram of our superficial and deep myofascia. In chapter 4, as you prepare to find trigger points in your body, you will see five of his diagrams so that you get the general idea of how tracts of fascia are organized (see figure 4.4, *a* through *e*). Seeing fascia in this way has helped many of our clients visualize the extent of fascial connections and how tightness or pain in one region may affect other regions along the same tract.

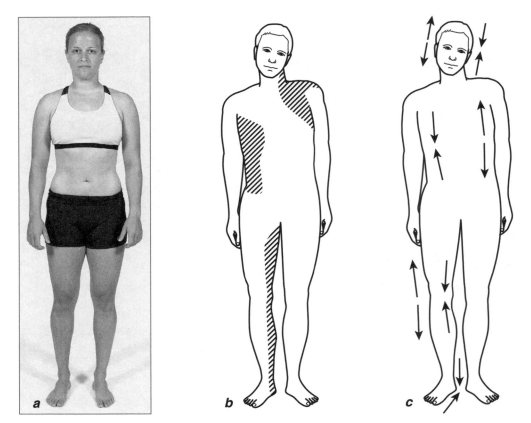

Figure 2.4 Compare relatively balanced posture (*a*), areas with stress and strain imbalances (*b*), the effects of such imbalances on the myofascia (*c*), and the postural asymmetrics related to the imbalances (*d*).

Compare the two postures in figure 2.4, *a* and *b*. In figure 2.4*b* you can see asymmetries in the tilt of the head, the lowered right shoulder, the high opposite hip, and the rotated right leg. Figure 2.4*c* shows how the myofascia under the skin might appear. If you then compare both the photo and the muscle drawing of the postural asymmetries with figure 2.4*d*, you may get an even better idea of the forces that become generated when posture gets imbalanced. With these comparative views, you are better able to visualize which muscle groups are shortened, tight, and compressed and which are lengthened, strained, and tense. When you study these figures you can visualize not only what is shortened and lengthened but also how the model's pattern presents as a logical, contiguous system of fascial stress and strain from head to feet. In chapter 4, you will be able to compare the asymmetries against the affected fascial lines. From these images you have a basis for predicting which areas will be shortened and tight under compression forces and which areas will be lengthened and tight under tensile forces. This is the way to start a critical analysis of flexibility. Studying your own posture can serve as a base from which to develop a full flexibility

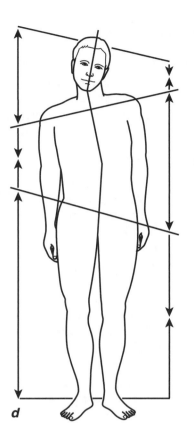

d

assessment, which we discuss in more detail in chapter 4.

When it comes to functional movement, you are still looking at posture, but now while in motion. Stress and strain can result from forces of tension and compression acting on or from within the body. This may be reflected in your posture and how tight or flexible you feel when you move. If you find when you examine your posture that you have a shorter leg on one side, you can imagine the impact this has on your walking or jumping. Without realizing it, perhaps in walking you tilt your trunk to avoid dragging or hitting your toe on the long-leg side. Or in jumping off two legs, you may notice that you favor one leg more than the other and that your takeoff and landing are not even. This kind of dynamic analysis often falls under the responsibility of coaches and trainers, who are constantly trying to sharpen their athletes' skills and techniques. If the movement error is due to technique, it will respond to coaching. If an athlete is not responding to coaching, however, then the perceptive coach knows that something in the body is not moving right, and the athlete needs to see the appropriate professional to get help for the problem.

Most of these asymmetries or errors of movement are due to pain or compensations. Compensations are what the body automatically does when it has to function with structural problems, as noted previously when we looked at postural asymmetry. A common example of compensatory movement caused by tight hips can be seen when an athlete does a squat incorrectly. For example, in a squat with good form, the legs are in alignment. But if the athlete has tight right hip external rotators, he or she is unable to keep the hip, knee, and foot aligned while performing the squat; the compensatory movement for the squat in this case is right hip external rotation, knee abduction, and foot pronation. If the athlete has trouble with proper alignment in this simple movement, you can be sure that it will show up in more complex movements as well and have a negative effect on performance. Consequently, you need to follow up postural analysis with functional movement analysis to get a comprehensive picture of what is going on within the body (see chapter 4).

Now that you know more about the structure of fascia, you can use this knowledge to better understand its function.

From Form to Fascial Function

As you learned in the previous section, the powerful combination of water's elastic tension with the plastic, elastic, and tensile properties of the ECM, elastin, and collagen makes your connective tissue system the premier target for stretching and increasing your flexibility. Before we show you the stretches, we describe how your connective tissue functions, specifically how your fascia functions. This will help you understand how you can improve much more than just your range of motion.

Again, think of the fascia as the body's internet, allowing for bodywide communication and embodying intelligence of movement. Recent biological discoveries have promoted the concept of sophisticated intelligence systems residing outside the brain in the body. For instance, science has recently classified a third nervous system (the central and autonomic systems being the other two) called the enteric nervous system, which appears to govern many functions of the digestive tract independent of the brain. Similarly, there is mounting evidence for independent roles played by the connective tissue system. One of our teachers and a colleague, James Oschman (2003), calls this system "the living matrix" because of its reach beyond the connective tissues and into "every organ, tissue, cell, molecule, atom, and subatomic particle within the body as well as the energy fields" that are within and around us. Because the connective tissue system has such extensive reach and influence, it offers great potential for improving much more than flexibility. We think that understanding the form and function of your fascia will help you realize that flexibility training is much more than just stretching. You will benefit on many levels besides flexibility when you stick with this system.

The integrity of the fascial net (that is, the connective tissue that is body wide and body deep, as well as the viscous environment it resides in, the ECM) depends on a system of physical and physiological balance. Physical balance is achieved by the mechanical design of the net and the efficient distribution of forces across it. The fascial net is a structure that has inherently balanced qualities of tension and integrity, or "tensegrity," a term coined by the engineer, great thinker, and inventor of the geodesic dome design, Buckminster Fuller. Figure 2.5, *a* and *b*, shows how the dome works. The dome has integrity because its structure

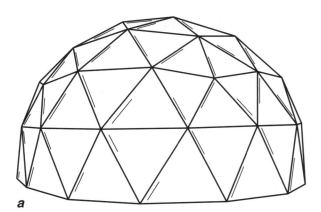

a

Figure 2.5 The freestanding geodesic dome (*a*) has tensegrity even when force is applied (*b*).

maintains its relative shape statically (when no forces other than gravity are exerted on it) and dynamically (when all kinds of forces are exerted on it). That is, it does not readily burst or break apart but "goes with the flow" to a great degree, efficiently distributing forces that would compress (stress) or pull (strain) it apart. After the forces are removed, it basically returns to the same shape it had before the forces were applied. Your body has an even better design in that it can instantly and simultaneously communicate to all the cells in your body through the structure of the fascial net how to move, change its shape, and adapt to the prevailing conditions. When you sit or lie down, your body adapts to the surface of the furniture or floor. But if you sit or stay in a position too long, your fascial system accumulates stress and strain from the summation of forces on the body and communicates to the mind and body that it must change position. If you do not change position often, as is the case with many who sit at work, then your fascia thickens in the areas that are under prolonged or repetitive stress and strain. This thickening is the body's automatic response to stress and strain in the myofascia. It is an attempt by the body to add extra strength to the tissue by depositing extra collagen. Unfortunately, this comes at the expense of flexibility; collagen alone is not the most flexible tissue, as anyone with a scar can attest.

Another example of the tensegrity of the fascial network is the way the body adapts to collision and extreme external pressure, such as that experienced by a running back in American football, who runs into human bodies and gets buried under a pile of them over and over again. As a result of tensegrity and flexibility, the running back's body automatically changes shape not only to cushion the blows but also to transmit the force of the blows and falls throughout the fascial network, just as the geodesic dome distributes forces throughout its structure. This helps to attenuate the magnitude of the forces so that they do not accumulate and overwhelm the involved tissue. Nevertheless, the body is programmed to deposit collagen in areas that are under repetitive stress and strain. Whether you are too inactive or extremely active in sports, the tendency of the body is to lay down extra collagen or scar tissue as an automatic reaction to stress and strain. The antidote, of course, is regular stretching. Stretching helps to realign collagen fibers that deposit themselves in a thick, disorganized manner. Stretching also creates length and space in the areas where collagen's effect has been to shorten and draw the tissue inward.

LOAD

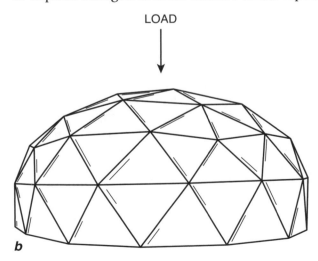

b

We just discussed how structural balance in the body is achieved by the mechanical design of the fascial net and by maintaining an efficient distribution of forces across it. Physiological balance of the body is also achieved by the mechanical design of the fascia.

The fascia has amazing physical and physiological integrity because it is designed to work synchronously with the muscles (as well as with every other structure and system) that it wraps around. That is why muscles and fascia are often referred to together as myofascia. Because of this intimate connection between muscle and fascia and because the fascial network is not only bodywide but also deep, the tone of muscle greatly influences the fascia and the state of the fascia greatly affects muscle tone.

Earlier in this chapter we discussed the division of a muscle into its smaller components, each successive component being defined, covered, and connected by the web of fascia it is also made of. All anatomical divisions—such as "muscle system" or "fascial system" —come from classical conventions for distinguishing items based on how they are named, categorized, or delineated. In truth, there is only one, unified and integrated functioning system that is more than the sum of its parts. Keeping this fact in mind may assist you in understanding how our physical form affects and is in turn affected by our physiological function. Figure 2.6 shows how the interconnected web of our connective tissue system specifically extends all the way down to the level of the cell by way of structures called integrins. Integrins contain collagen and play a physical and physiological role in the attachment of a cell to the ECM and in communication (signal transduction) between the ECM and the cell. They do this at least partially by transferring information about physical movement to and from the connective tissue of the cell. Physical movement—either cell movement, as when our skin migrates to heal internal or external wounds, or whole body movement, as when we run or jump—in turn influences the biochemical and biophysical reactions that occur in cells, tissues, organs and systems.

As a result of the extent of the fascial web, reaching from the level of the skin all the way in to the deepest cells of the body, when any part of the body moves, whether voluntarily or involuntarily, all the cells get this mechanical message of movement as it undulates and reverberates through the fascial network at the speed of light (Oschman 2003). Think about how quickly you can react, correct your movement, and avoid a serious injury when you have missed a step while walking downstairs or thought that there was another step when going upstairs. We have all had this type of experience, but do we really understand the implications of it? You use this ability to react and adjust every day, but you especially depend on it in sports for superior performance and to protect yourself from getting hurt. What makes it possible is rapid communication throughout the bodywide web of connective tissue, which simultaneously communicates with other systems such as the nervous and circulatory systems, stimulating the activation of nerve impulses as well as hormonal secretions, among many other things.

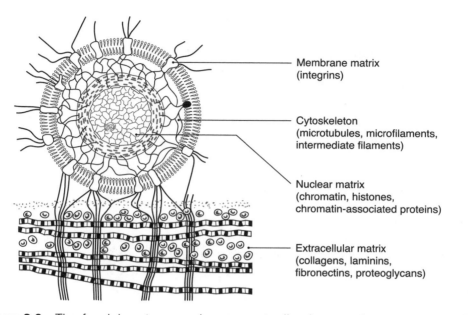

Figure 2.6 The fascial system can be conceptualized as continuous, structurally and physiologically connecting the muscle belly to the cells. In this figure, wavy lines of collagen from the extracellular matrix connect to the cytoskeleton by way of the integrins.

Reprinted from *Energy medicine: The scientific basis*, J. Oschman, p. 66, 2000, with permission from Elsevier.

If your myofascial system has faults in it such as scar tissue, tightness, or trigger points, then it cannot optimally communicate and cooperate with the other systems of your body. Consequently, your athletic execution is less than optimal and you may hear a coach remark that you "just are not flowing today!"

Simply put, the physiology might go something like this: The fascial system gets tight from any number of causes (see pages 31 to 33), which decreases the circulatory system's ability to supply blood since it travels through the fascia, which in turn decreases blood supply to the working muscles. For most athletes and coaches, early fatigue, soreness or sometimes even pain, is not an acceptable reason to stop training. So an athlete will continue training through those symptoms, most often without even letting the coach know about them. This results in increased muscle tension, or tone. By *tone*, we mean the muscle is in a relative state of physiological activity but not necessarily contracting. Physiological activity could be anything from cellular metabolism in the muscle to low-level bioelectrical activity that does not lead to muscle contraction, to the undulating ebb and flow of air in the lungs and fluids in the body that are gently moving the myofascia with every breath, heartbeat, and pulse of spinal fluid. Muscle tone is what maintains a consistent shape in the connective tissue. When you are sleeping you have low muscle tone, or low activation; when you are lifting weights you have high muscle tone, or high activation.

A tight fascial system leads to higher muscle tone because it increases the output from the nervous system required to initiate and perform movements, both to prime mover muscles and to the secondary and tertiary muscles that may have to help the prime movers. We see this with our football clients, who can still run when they have higher muscle tone, but use more energy and have a running style that is inefficient and lacks flow. Although this may work for athletes in the short term, they are overtraining their muscles and will start using other, less efficient patterns of movement because of working through what becomes a chronic cycle of pain, soreness, and tightness. These undesirable patterns of movement are called *compensations* because they compensate for what the athletes lack, such as flexibility, by using other movements to perform an action. Otherwise, they don't get to play or train when the pressure is on. Naturally, when an athlete is having these difficulties, he or she gets increasingly frustrated. Something that used to come easily is now hard work, and it hurts too! At this point the athlete no longer is able to stay in the "zone" and his or her movement is no longer flowing. Sound familiar? This is often what happens just before a season- or even a career-ending injury.

Muscle tone is automatically set and regulated by the central nervous system in the part of the brain called the cerebellum as well as in other areas of the brain and spinal cord. The cerebellum also performs a number of other motor and cognitive functions, including motor learning, movement planning, motor timing, posture maintenance, and some cognitive and attentive functions—in other words, everything you rely on in sports. Therefore, because everything in the body works in feedback loops, improving your muscle tone improves the function of your brain, which in turn improves athletic performance.

Even though your postural muscles are automatically regulated by the central nervous system, your muscle tone is always being modulated by the autonomic nervous system (ANS). The ANS is responsible for homeostasis, maintaining a relatively constant internal environment by controlling such involuntary functions as digestion, respiration, perspiration, and metabolism and by modulating blood pressure. Although these functions are generally beyond conscious control, they are not beyond your awareness, and they may be influenced by your state of mind, which obviously is affected by the state of your body.

The autonomic nervous system is divided into the sympathetic nervous system (SNS) and the parasympathetic nervous system (PNS). The SNS and PNS work together in both synchronous and antagonistic ways. When you are active and engaged in sports, you are functioning primarily with the SNS. When you are relaxing or sleeping, you are functioning with the PNS. The SNS activates skeletal muscles for action and therefore stimulates muscle tone to be relatively high, or hypertonic. When you rely on the PNS, muscle tone is low, or hypotonic. When you work out or train, your muscles swell with extra blood flow based on the demands imposed. Because connective tissue has elastic qualities, it allows the muscles to contract and expand with heavy exertion. If you work your muscles to failure or extreme fatigue, you get the familiar increase in tone accompanied by pain or soreness and stiffness 24 to 48 hours later. This may be caused by a variety of elements, such as microtearing of muscle fibers, increased waste products in the blood from increased activity, and increased collagen production by the connective tissue to heal what was stressed or strained. We have seen time and time again that if our clients are doing heavy weight training, trying to put on extra body mass, or simply training or playing very hard in their sports, their myofascia becomes increasingly tight and they lose their flexibility. Their muscle tone increases and the elastic quality of their tissue decreases. Fortunately, you can do heavy training without losing flexibility in the process; in later chapters we show you how. The point is that your body structure will change for the better or worse based on the design of your training program. So the elements of the program must be balanced and individualized in order for your body to function optimally. Proper program design is covered in chapter 5.

In the next section we identify common factors that can negatively affect your flexibility. We then offer solutions for the challenges posed by those factors.

Factors Affecting Flexibility

Many factors can influence how your body and mind feel and function, but we focus on the two most common factors that affect your flexibility and stretching based on our clinical and personal experience: physical and mental or emotional factors.

Physical

We have seen three common physical factors that contribute to inflexibility or a feeling of tightness: simple muscle tension from poor posture, the many ways that the body has compensated for injuries, and positions an athlete repeatedly assumes for his or her sport. These three factors are actually interdependent, but we explain them separately in order to understand how they work together.

Good posture is generally understood by athletes and fit people as standing or sitting erect and not slouching. We take it a few steps further so that you understand the relationship between posture and flexibility. For the purpose of this book, we define good posture as the most efficient way to be in command of your body so that it serves your purpose without pain and unnecessary stress or strain. This is generally attained when all the structures of your body are in balanced alignment with regard to gravity and each other. You can maintain this balance, once you have achieved it, by performing activities that help balance one another. For example, if you are doing a lot of strength work in weightlifting, perhaps to gain more mass, then you must balance it with a lot of stretching. Or, if you work at a job where you sit all day, then you must balance it with more standing activities. When the structures of the body are not balanced this way, then stress and strain, by way of forces generating myofascial compression and tension, develop and begin to change your balanced alignment.

Stress and strain may come from either too much activity (overtraining) or too little activity (undertraining). When these kinds of forces develop in the body, the body functions differently in order to adapt to and accommodate the stress and strain. Over time these forces are chronically present, and the only way the body knows how to deal with constant extra forces is to deposit more collagen (scar tissue) for support. The deposit of extra collagen upsets the balance of elastin, water, and other elements that gives your tissues mobility and flexibility, tilting it in the direction of increased rigidity in tissues. An additional manifestation of stress and strain is in the development of firm, tender nodules in myofascia, commonly called *knots* by athletes and *trigger points* by clinicians. Trigger points are a source of pain, soreness, tightness, and stiffness locally and generally. As a result of extra collagen deposits, trigger points, and the uncomfortable symptoms previously noted, the body's fascial web starts to distort the position and shape, seen both on the inside as well as the outside of your body. Outwardly, this is seen as changes in your posture as parts of your body bend, shift, and rotate in response to the accumulation of the forces of stress and strain previously described. Some parts of your fascia shorten in response to compressive loads and other parts excessively lengthen in response to tensile loads. In either case, collagen is deposited in these areas and reduces your overall flexibility.

Injuries from some time ago can be a cause of present-day pain or tightness, which can inhibit an athlete's ability to stretch efficiently. Although the original injury may have healed, the patterns that the athlete's body formed to compensate for it may still exist. For example, an old ankle sprain may still manifest itself as a compensatory presence in a shortened, externally rotated leg. This pattern commonly starts right after the sprain, when in an effort to protect and stabilize the leg while walking the person demonstrates a bit of a "peg leg" gait. Over time, the pattern more or less remains, even though the person no longer has ankle pain. In fact, it appears that the more time has passed since the original incident, the more the compensations distribute themselves throughout the body—often-times far from the original injury. In response to the externally rotated leg, for example, it is common for the body to rotate the pelvis or ribs in the opposite direction as a compensation pattern of position and movement.

While compensations take on some predictable patterns, they are also highly individual and reflect the activities that a person engages in. For example, the effects of an externally rotated leg may have fewer implications for a ballet dancer who already spends all her time moving her hips that way than for a long-distance cyclist who must keep his hips and legs parallel for long periods in the saddle. In either case, the altered patterns are usually the result of the body's taking the path of least resistance rather than the path of greatest efficiency in movement. This causes the body to do more work than is necessary, which again leads to increased stress and strain and all the associated negative changes that go along with that. Over time, the compensations accumulate and create a vicious cycle of stress, strain, tightness, and pain so that efficient, flowing movement is no longer possible and the athlete must step away from the sport. Through the Stretch to Win system we teach you how to identify and correct compensations so that they do not impede your progress on the road to efficient stretching and optimal flexibility.

Habitual functional postures are yet another factor contributing to specific or overall inflexibility. An example of a functional posture that is habitual is the baseball catcher's position. Years of playing in the catcher's severely crouched position take their toll on the back, hips, and knees, especially when he does not perform daily stretches of the specific areas that get chronically tight from assuming this position. Despite what the body does to heal and recover from each day's activity, patterns of strain often remain and accumulate in the body's myofascia. This may be apparent in the form of chronic aches and pains or a feeling of general or specific tightness. Unfortunately, the athlete usually blames these feelings on years of playing and starts to rely on medications to get through training and playing. Over time, the athlete develops the compensations to deal with this tightness, as discussed previously, and these become primary problems that contribute to fascial distortions and postural imbalances. These imbalances may be the result of how the athlete makes adjustments because of decreased speed, power, or strength. By working with athletes in their formative years, we can help them develop good habits of training and avoid this scenario.

Mental and Emotional Factors

We mentioned that physical stress and strain distort the body's fascia, which in turn causes more stress and strain. Naturally, functioning in a body that is no longer pain free and efficient at moving catalyzes mental and emotional reactions. A bad mood or attitude resulting in crankiness and lack of cooperation can progress over time to feelings of depression and hopelessness. Because many of us have experienced this vicious cycle, we probably have taken medications to make the physical symptoms go away. Unfortunately, this only masks the symptoms, because medications do not cure the problem of scar tissue. As a result, the liver gets stressed for many years as it tries to filter and detoxify the drugs in the body.

Different people handle day-to-day stress differently, and attentive coaches and trainers know that stress needs to be addressed on an individual basis. For athletes, it pays to get to know how their bodies react to mental or emotional stress so that they can address at least some aspect of it on the physical level, thereby decreasing some of the negative effects of stress on the body. Those athletes who feel excessively on edge whether in training or in competition need to find ways to alleviate this stress to get the most out of their performance as well as to get the most out of the rest period immediately postactivity. We have found that a very effective way to manage stress in such athletes is to use regular stretching with synchronized breathing to keep excessive tension from developing in the muscles. Managing mental and emotional stress this way directs at least a measure of help to conserve precious energy resources, decrease compensatory patterns of movement from unnecessary myofascial tension, and decrease the risk of injury from poor concentration.

chapter 3

Flexibility for Sport Performance

I n the previous chapter you learned that your fascia is a highly responsive material that adapts and changes to prevailing conditions, and that it will give you fewer problems if you keep it in a state of balance. You also began to learn how to recognize the telltale signs of flexibility problems by analyzing posture and some functional positions. This chapter helps you identify more of these signs by evaluating the way you feel and move, thereby giving you insight into your athletic performance as well as your flexibility. We cover common structural indicators of flexibility as well as other indicators you can observe in your functional movements in both sports and ordinary activities of daily living.

When a lack of mobility or stability prevents you from performing a daily activity normally, you develop compensations of movement to adapt to the restrictions and still perform the task. These compensations carry over to the more advanced movements you use in athletic activities.

Structural Factors

We see three common structural conditions in our clinic that indicate problems with flexibility. Often the underlying causes of limitations to movement are hypomobile joint capsules, scar tissue in the myofascia, and trigger points in the myofascia.

- **Hypomobile joint capsules.** As we stated in chapter 1, nearly 50 percent of a healthy person's lack of range of motion at the joint can be attributed to the tightness of the joint capsule. Because the joint capsule often shares its innervation with the muscles that cross over it, these muscles respond by getting tight or hypertonic. Of course, the opposite sequence can happen as well, when the muscle gets injured and forms scar tissue, causing the joint capsule to respond by tightening and restricting range of motion. In either case, the outcome is the same—a hypomobile joint.

How can you tell if one of your joints is hypomobile? When you focus your movement on a hypomobile joint, you will usually feel an abrupt block to the movement. You may experience this if you try to kneel by sitting in the traditional Japanese position, with your knees maximally flexed and resting on the ground, your lower legs folded under your thighs, and your feet pointed down so that the tops of your feet are on the ground while your bottom rests on your heels. Hypomobile knee and ankle joint capsules can make it difficult to get into this position. On the other hand, if you cannot get down properly into full squat position when weightlifting, your hip joint capsules (along with your psoas muscle) may be blocking your attempts. In limiting your range of motion, hypomobile joints can also reduce your strength. To use the squat as an example again, if hypomobile hip joints prevent you from dropping down into the end position of the squat movement, you will not get the stretch of the glutes to assist you in lowering and lifting the weight. This problem is even more pronounced in the case of a power squat, which requires a quick stretch of the quads, glutes, and low back fascia to help you explode out of that deep position. A hypomobile joint, then, can reduce the speed and power of your movements.

- **Scar tissue.** Collagen in the form of scar tissue in muscle and fascia is very common. As we explained in chapter 2, the body deposits collagen in any region that is under stress or strain in an attempt to strengthen tissues by thickening them. This can occur both when you overtrain and when you undertrain. Excessive strenuous exertion, such as when American football players try to put on extra muscle mass in the off-season, will make an athlete tighter because of increased stress and strain in the fascia. We see the results of overtraining all the time in our clinic. On the other hand, if an athlete takes too long a break from training, he or she will feel not only weaker but also tighter from not moving enough. Physically not moving much or being inactive can also be a source of stress and strain, and the body responds to it by depositing scar tissue. Extra collagen in the form of scar tissue in your body slows you down in sports and in activities of daily living, because tissue with extra collagen loses some of its elasticity. This is where stretching comes in, helping you to recover and maintain your elasticity despite the stress and strain of training, competition, and injury.

- **Trigger points.** Trigger points, which can be caused by a multitude of factors, are a major and common cause of myofascial pain and dysfunction. They may exist anywhere in our connective tissue, in fascia, muscles, ligaments, bones, and even fat (Travell 1983). In muscles they manifest as firm, tender nodules commonly known as knots. Usually when you put pressure on a trigger point the pain radiates outward a fair distance, and you may feel like there is pressure on a nerve. You might find the exact location of a trigger point in your muscle when you instinctively poke around in an area, like at the back of the base of your neck and shoulder, and feel a large tender knot that sends pain down your shoulder blade or arm. But if you do not press on the trigger point, you may not even know it's there until you attempt some movement such as raising your arm overhead and find you can't do it because of pain in your shoulder. If you completely rely on your arms and shoulders, as swimmers, pitchers, and basketball players do, trigger points in this area can give you great trouble, making your arm seem to shut down in the middle of a movement and causing you to lose trust and confidence in using it. Trigger points can both tighten and weaken muscles, causing painful restrictions of movement. Your essential athletic abilities—such as strength, power, speed, quickness, and agility—can be compromised, all because of a silly trigger point!

Fortunately, you can avoid, eliminate, or greatly reduce all three of these conditions by assessing and treating them before they develop into problems. You will learn how to do this in the next chapter. In the meantime, we will look at how these factors affect your flexibility and movement.

Functional Movement Indicators

Success in sports often comes down to an athlete's ability to skillfully direct power and agility as a means to an end. Whether that end is a championship game, an Olympic record, or a sincere effort to push one's limits by training with a coach, premium athleticism depends on effective training. Apart from the variety of specialized training approaches available today, there are fundamental movements in everyday life that athletes should monitor to make sure they are meeting their flexibility goals.

The training for any activity that involves movement can be organized into a pyramid in which functional movement is at the base, functional performance is in the middle, and functional skill is at the top (figure 3.1; see Cook 2003

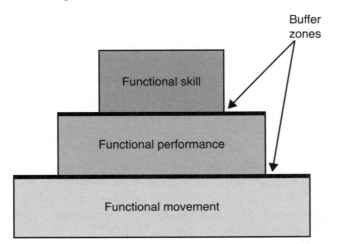

Figure 3.1 Cook's performance pyramid illustrates the importance of a solid foundation.
Reprinted, by permission, from G. Cook, 2003, *Athletic body in balance* (Champaign, IL: Human Kinetics), 13.

for more on this paradigm). To achieve excellence in sports performance and athletic skills, you must build them on a solid foundation of functional movement and power. Although many athletes are able to perform at the functional skill level without having solid functional movement skills, we have seen that they are not able to continue at that level; often this becomes apparent in rehabilitation after they sustain injuries.

Athletic Movements

Ideally, an athlete should have a balanced training program to condition his or her body for sport performance. This means that the preseason, in-season, postseason, and off-season work should be balanced to help the athlete achieve optimal flexibility, strength, power, agility, endurance, and sport-specific skills at the right time and in the right order. If the progression is not optimal, the athlete may become overtrained or undertrained, with either situation creating a poor state of preparedness. A gifted athlete may still perform at a very high level in one of these situations, but usually not for any appreciable length of time before stress and strain develop in the soft tissues, eventually resulting in some type of injury. While injuries may still happen to an athlete who is optimally prepared, much research suggests that certain training progression protocols reduce injuries, which is one reason that virtually every high school, college, and professional team follows some sort of training program system. A complete program of strength and conditioning for athletes is beyond the scope of this book, but in chapter 5 we discuss how to fit a flexibility program into the context of the rest of your sport training and conditioning.

If your training incorporates the three principles noted in figure 3.1, then you have the basis for a proper training progression. The bottommost principle, functional movement, is the first element of that progression. One of our favorite responses to athletes who ask us when they will be ready to start running again after an injury is "When your walking is effortless and efficient." The way you walk, an example of functional movement, is indicative of so many aspects of athleticism. Yes, it is possible for an athlete to have an inefficient gait and even a little pain on one side with every step and still perform at an elite level. However, this athlete's days of athletic effectiveness are numbered—sooner or later, cumulative stress and strain will take him or her down. Functional movements, the ones that we all learned as children through trial and error with our parents' encouragement and that we engage in every day, are supposed to be effortless, energy efficient, and pain free. This means that going through position changes—from standing to sitting to getting on the floor to looking under the bed and so on—should all be easy and painless.

Activities of Daily Living

Activities of daily living (ADLs) are the physical activities that adults do daily but often take for granted, such as dressing, cleaning, and playing with children. If you find yourself struggling to put on your socks or tie your shoes because of a decreased range of motion, you should "red flag" the moments as warning signs—these limitations will also affect your athletic performance. If optimal athletic performance requires that movement be effective and efficient under the most demanding conditions, then it stands to reason that movement should be this way at all times. When it is not, over time your body habituates to the adjustments it has to make. In other words, you get used to moving with compensations.

To use a common illustration of this effect, the most efficient path to take when you want to walk or run from one point to another is along a straight line. If there are obstacles in this path, you have to take a detour to get to your destination. This detour adds more time to the trip and consequently requires more energy expenditure. Similarly, when the body takes detours to make a movement happen, it uses more time and energy to accomplish the movement. For example, if you kneel on one knee to retrieve an object from the floor and your upright knee moves inward instead of directly over the foot below it, then it is taking a detour that is less efficient and harder work for the knee joint and muscles. In such cases the stress to your joints and strain to your muscles, tendons, and ligaments contribute to future incorrect patterns of movement.

The simple movements of ADL involve transitions from one position to another that you learned as a developing child. The correct patterns of these movements, such as changing from a sitting position to a standing one, become part of your daily movement vocabulary and serve as a reference for all sorts of other movements. If something happens to interrupt a child's normal development of these fundamental patterns, a less efficient compensatory movement pattern can remain throughout life, unless some sort of movement reeducation or physical therapy is successfully undertaken. For example, the ability to squat efficiently is usually first gained in childhood. But if you never fully achieved this in childhood, you will probably always have difficulty correctly assuming the squat position for any sport or training that requires it, unless you eliminate your compensations and retrain for efficiency of movement.

As an adult, you may start to develop movement compensations in response to tightness or new or old injuries without knowing that this is happening. The way you perform your ADLs can provide you with the first telltale signs of subtle problems that may grow into bigger ones under the stress of athletic activities. The "weekend warriors" come to mind, going all out in competitive games like basketball and tennis, and getting injured or sore as a result of their bodies getting way out of balance.

As another example, let's examine how one ADL—putting on your socks—can reveal issues that might affect athletic movement. Perhaps you find that it is not an easy task to put on either sock but that the right one gives you more trouble in the form of hip pain or tightness. Some people prefer to put on their socks while standing and others while sitting. To do it standing requires good balance, stability on the standing leg, and adequate mobility of the moving leg. To do it sitting requires adequate flexion in the trunk and hip to bring the thigh to the chest (or the chest to the thigh). If you cannot perform these simple movements because of restrictions or pain in the back or hip, then you will develop other ways to put on a sock. These other ways are adaptations or compensations for a lack of ability to perform what should be a simple daily activity. Most of us prefer to follow the path of least resistance rather than struggle with a more difficult movement (you are, after all, just putting on your socks), but your abilities will remain restricted if you never address the problem. If your ADLs demonstrate that you have tight hips, and if your sport requires hip flexibility, you should be aware that you will compensate in even greater ways during athletic activity because of the added intensity, power, and speed that are required for most sports movements.

For instance, if you are performing full squats with weights in training, it will be difficult to maintain good form—stable and erect back and symmetrical pelvis-hip-knee-foot angles—if your hips feel tight when you're just putting on your socks. Compounding the problem of tightness by adding weights (intensity), repetitions (frequency), and sets (duration) eventually leads to greater compensations, which turn into habits that are difficult to break, even with coaching. As this all-too-common scenario builds over time, a chronic state of stress, strain, and pain when you work out or compete leads you to think that this is normal and that the burning and aching you feel are OK. This might be an effective way to operate if burning calories were the only goal. But in terms of efficiency of movement, the production and use of energy, and cumulative training effects, it is a dismal failure. Many athletes are drawn into this cycle, as evidenced by the habitual use of knee and elbow braces, elasticized bandages, and medications for pain and inflammation. While there are medically indicated uses for these modalities, they are often used inappropriately as a crutch by those who have not addressed their underlying movement imbalances and compensations.

Improving your basic movement patterns and abilities in your ADLs will lay down the groundwork for your more complex athletic training. When you become accustomed to periodically checking in with how your body is feeling and performing from the time you wake up until the time you go to sleep, you can evaluate and treat small problems before they become big ones. These brief, daily self-assessments increase your self-awareness and keep you at an optimal level of functioning, helping you meet the demands you put on your body and mind. We teach you how to perform them in chapter 4.

Core Strength

Over the last 50 years, many researchers in the fields of medicine, physical rehabilitation, and physical therapy have studied the neuromuscular effects of conditions such as polio, muscular dystrophy, and stroke. These effects can include loss of strength, flexibility, balance, and overall motor control. The research has shown that before patients can regain functional mobility of their arms and legs, they must reacquire good stabilizing strength in the central, or core, region of the body—the abdominal, gluteal, and back muscles. This confirms what is seen in human infant motor development; babies must first strengthen their

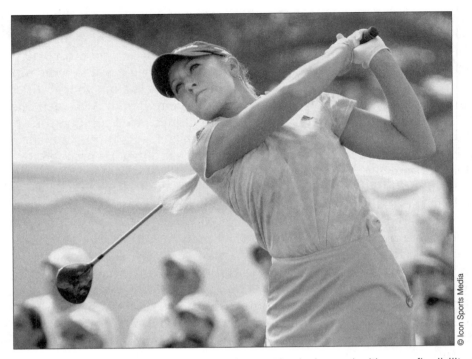

© Icon Sports Media

In all forms of athletic activity, core strength must be balanced with core flexibility to achieve optimal performance.

cores before they can learn to crawl and then walk. In recent years, interest in strengthening the core muscle groups of the trunk and pelvis has grown in most areas of sports and fitness. It's been found that this training can lead to gains in an athlete's balance, coordination, and agility as well as strength, power, and endurance.

Most programs of physical training today incorporate some form of core strengthening or core conditioning. The best programs recognize that in a normal child's development the trunk and pelvis are naturally trained over a predictable period of time, in a familiar sequence of progressive movements that are learned by trial and error. That is, eventually the child learns how to activate the core musculature, not by receiving special coaching or by doing isolated core strengthening exercises, but by making mistakes before *experiencing what feels right and what makes a movement work.* Probably one of the more visible examples of this, besides an infant lifting the head for the first time, is when an infant learns to roll from the back to the belly. After many unsuccessful attempts, one day the baby figures out the right way to recruit the core muscles and coordinate them with the mobility of the limbs and succeeds. From that moment on, the infant remembers how to coordinate stability before mobility. The growing child progresses through each advanced movement challenge, learning to walk, run, and play sports with naturally developed core strength and stability.

Until the body succumbs to immobility, disease, or injury, its innate intelligence remembers how to activate the core. Since research in physical medicine and physical therapy first showed a faster and more complete return to function when rehabilitation included core postural education and strength training, core work is now found outside of rehab and in virtually every athletic strength and conditioning training program. The best programs help you develop the ability to activate your core muscles without thinking, at the moment, they are needed so that you can be safely and effectively mobile.

In most cases, you must have a stable core to produce the most efficient movement. The following test helps illustrate this (do not try this if you have a current condition of pain). Lie flat on your back with both legs lying straight in front of you on the floor. First lift the right leg about a foot off the floor or ground and note how light or heavy it feels and how much your pelvis twists or rotates in response to lifting it. Now return the leg to the starting position and repeat with the left leg. Note any changes in how the leg, hip, pelvis, and back feel and whether the lift feels smoother or more effortless on one side than on the other. If you have an imbalance, you may notice on the side that does not feel right that the lifted leg feels heavier and that the pelvis and back twist or rotate more, producing a feeling of a lack of stability or support. If you experience lack of stability or support, then it is likely that you have some core activation problems.

Targeted stretching of the correct muscle groups can help release core strength when inhibition is the cause of weakness. For instance, tight hip flexors will inhibit the gluteals from activating and then may act in place of the core to attempt to provide stability when the main core muscles of the trunk, pelvis, and hips should be the dominant players. Stretching the hip flexors often eliminates this problem. If core activation still poses a problem, you will want to go to a professional who has a good reputation in core retraining. This person should perform a full evaluation and come up with a plan to address the problem. Targeted stretching is just one way flexibility training can become part of an integrated approach to bringing the body into balance.

Balanced Mobility and Stability

In the previous section about core strength, we pointed out that babies must first strengthen their core muscles before they can learn to crawl and then walk. In physical therapy we denote this same concept by saying generally that stability must be present in order for normal mobility to occur. Normal mobility, for the purposes of this particular discussion, refers to the ability of a person to move any part of his or her body, using the joints and muscles, without pain or restriction. This movement is accomplished with a balance of mobility and stability.

An example would be the simple act of lifting your hand up to change a light bulb that is on the ceiling. Imagine that you go up a little on the balls of your feet as you stretch your shoulder joint and muscles to reach the bulb. If you have normal mobility in your shoulder that is balanced with stability, this chore is simple and pain free. If you are tight in your shoulder, you can perhaps still perform the action with good stability, but your mobility is associated with a pulling or stretching sensation of a greater or lesser magnitude, depending on how tight you are and where you are tight. If you are looser in the shoulder joint than the average person, then even though you can perform the action using sufficient range of motion, you may strain the joint. You may feel pain, discomfort, or lack of strength in holding up the arm, depending on how and where you lack stability in the muscles coupled with where and how loose you are in the joints of your shoulder complex.

Normal mobility may be viewed as a range; on one end of the normal range are people who have slightly looser joints and on the other end are people who have slightly tighter joints. In physical therapy and other fields, looser than normal joints are called hypermobile and tighter than normal joints are called hypomobile; both are considered abnormal states that require some form of treatment if they affect optimal function. These states of increased or decreased movement in the structure of the body may exist in whole or in part. That is, in some people all of the connective tissue in the body is slightly looser than normal, while in others all of the connective tissue is slightly tighter than average. Still others may be looser in the upper body and tighter in the lower body. Some people may have only one shoulder that is very loose while the rest of the body is average in flexibility. In reality, it may be more accurate to view your body as having its own range of tightness on one end of the scale and looseness on the other, to account for the variety of flexibility that is found within the body. This view helps you see and work with your specific needs—flexibility and otherwise—when it comes to preparing for improved performance.

In this book, we are only considering a bell curve of normal joint and muscle range of motion (see *Manual Muscle Testing* by Florence Kendall for a complete list of numerical joint ranges), with normal being in the center of the curve and those who are slightly above (or slightly hypermobile) and slightly below the average (or slightly hypomobile) at the ends of the curve. Classifications for what is considered normal range of motion for joints and the muscles that cross them are varied, depending on the source, and are even controversial. Therefore in order to keep it simple but still accurate and logical, we suggest that you use the previous example of changing a light bulb as one simple guideline to help you evaluate what you feel when you move; if the movement is easy and pain free, all is well. Keep in mind that different body regions have specific ranges of flexibility—you'll gain a better understanding of your body's idiosyncrasies when you master doing your own personal flexibility assessment in chapter 4. While only an experienced practitioner, such as a licensed physical therapist or other professional, can come up with an accurate diagnosis of a particular problem or pain, using the simple guidelines given in this book will help you improve your flexibility and athletic performance.

When we train students in our school, we often get the question, "Is it OK to stretch muscles that cross an already hypermobile or loose joint?" If you are involved in a sport or activity that requires more than a "normal" range of motion to successfully participate, yes, you absolutely need to stretch to attain and then maintain that hypermobility. For example, a pitcher must have much more external range of motion in the shoulder for his sport than he needs for his activities of daily living. Yet along with that extra motion there must also be localized stability and strength to support the extra motion, or an unstable joint will result.

Instability usually refers to joints that have lax ligaments, which can be caused by previous injury (sprain) to the area. Instability can also arise when excessive stretching or sport-skill training (like pitching) results in hypermobility of the joint and muscles of the region but is not balanced with sufficient strengthening. For example, Mary A. was a client in her 50s who had been a serious yoga practitioner for 30 years. She came to us to be stretched because she felt tight and had discomfort in her low back. When we evaluated her, we determined that she was generally hypermobile in her joints and was bordering on instability in many of her weight-bearing joints. Also, her general muscle tone was lower than it should have been. When we tested her strength we determined that she was very weak in her core muscle groups of the trunk, pelvis, and hips. We put her on a core strengthening and stabilization routine; within two weeks her back pain was resolved. Mary did not need stretching, she needed strengthening. You can avoid instability by engaging in a balanced program of strengthening and stabilization exercises for hypermobile joints.

On the other end of the continuum is hypomobility. The best thing for joints and muscles that have restrictions to their range of movement is stretching. In chapter 1, as you may remember, principle 7 is "Target the entire joint" and principle 8 is "Use traction for maximal lengthening." Athletes who have hypomobile joints and tight myofascia get the most dramatic gains from stretching, because it releases all the locked-up potential in the joint capsule and fascia. Liberating that movement opens the door to maximal performance.

Functional Performance and Flexibility

As noted in figure 3.1, the next tier of athletic training is functional performance, in which the athlete trains to improve his or her strength, speed, power, agility, and endurance. Of course, as you know from reading the previous sections, if an athlete moves to this level without first mastering the fundamentals of functional movement, he or she will have problems. If these fundamentals are not mastered, compensations in movement will develop. For example, if an athlete lacks good core control he or she will overwork the extremities, resulting in unnecessary stress and strain. When training includes advanced power moves such as plyometric jumps, fatigue and failure will occur much sooner with a weak, poorly activated core muscle group.

Optimal functional performance in sports depends on optimal training in strength, power, speed, agility, quickness, balance, and endurance. All of these parameters can be negatively affected if you do not also have optimal flexibility in your fascial system. Remember that because your fascia intertwines with and covers your muscles, nerves, and bones, any change in the state of any of these systems affects all the other systems.

Strength

The late movement scientist and biomechanist Mel Siff, PhD, created the classic definition of strength, "the ability of a given muscle or group of muscles to generate muscular force under specific conditions." He also said that strength is not primarily a function of muscle size but rather of whether the appropriate muscles are powerfully contracted by effective nervous stimulation. This is the foundation of all strength training. In sports, strength training is a necessary part of preparing the athlete to perform at his or her maximum. Anything that detracts from strength or from the functioning of the nervous system, therefore, will not allow maximum athletic performance. A lack of flexibility is one factor that can inhibit strength.

For example, think of how mental or emotional stress can cause increased tension in your nervous system. As we discuss in chapter 2, the central nervous system is responsible for muscle tone. Muscle tone is labile—that is, it changes as it responds to internal and external stimuli. When you are stressed, your muscle tone increases. This may be temporary, as when you hear a loud noise and duck, or it may be chronic, as it is for many of the athlete clients who come to our clinic. Having unnecessary tension in your myofascia is like wearing a long-sleeve shirt and pants that are two sizes too small for you—much too tight! This tightness can slow the movement of nutrients into your tissues and of waste products out of them, because hypertonic myofascia often constricts blood vessels. This decreases the efficiency of muscles' recovery from both aerobic and anaerobic activity and thus decreases strength and endurance. Keeping your myofascia mobile will optimize nutrient facilitation, waste elimination, and an entire array of body functions for better physical performance.

Speed

Speed is also known as velocity. Intuitively, you know that when you feel tight you cannot move as quickly or efficiently as you can when you are looser. It is the absence of the feeling of tightness that we are trying to achieve in the Stretch to Win system. We should qualify our use of the word "loose," which, in our experience in speaking with athletes, has several meanings that are actually distinct from simply the opposite of "tight." The idea is not to feel loose in the sense of unstable or too flexible, but rather to have complete freedom of movement with no restrictions when you train and compete.

The professional football players we work with often describe tightness as feeling like their parking brakes have been put on when they attempt to run at full speed on the field. Sometimes the tightness makes them fear they will pull a hamstring and they decide not to run at maximum capacity. Despite great coaching, they find themselves unable to get their speed up to their potential. Their coaches may start to think that they are lazy or not trying hard enough, and the athletes get frustrated that they cannot perform at their maximum.

Increasing flexibility can increase speed by helping the athlete feel at his or her best. Typical responses from our clients after stretching using our system are that they feel lighter and are able to move with more freedom. Record-breaking football player Emmitt Smith, now retired, said after his first session, "It made me feel like I am 10 years younger." This is a common response from our veteran players, because the system helps them perform with more speed and agility than they may have had in years.

Power

In biomechanics power is the product of force (strength) and velocity over a specific range of motion around a joint or joints. Scientists use calculus, computer-generated models, and multiple video cameras to analyze the complexities of movement. All we are concerned with here, however, is that your ability to generate force is decreased if your muscles tighten up from trigger points, scar tissue, joint hyper- or hypomobility, or other causes. If you cannot generate the appropriate amount of force, you cannot increase your velocity. Consequently, power production goes down on all counts. Increased tightness from any cause will decrease your power.

For example, if you have a trigger point in a muscle, according to noted authority and researcher Janet Travel, MD, the muscle becomes hypertonic and hyperirritable, and generally possesses a lowered threshold to external and internal stimulation. In a power move such as pitching a baseball, a trigger point in the rotator cuff could cause a misfiring of muscle fibers when the cuff is activated. This could lead to decreased ball velocity, poor target accuracy, and early fatigue, among other problems. A trigger point demonstrates an altered

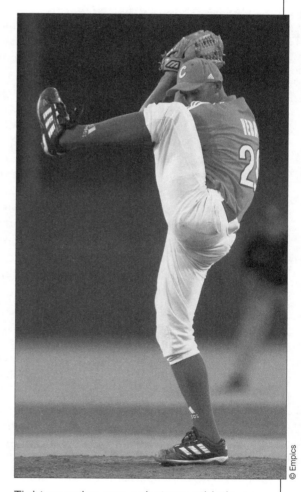

© Empics

Tight muscles can sabotage athletic performance by reducing power, interfering with accuracy, and decreasing overall endurance.

metabolism—most notably ischemic hypoxia or a lower oxygen content in the muscle because local blood flow is too low—it will also decrease endurance in athletes like marathoners, distance swimmers, and cyclists.

Agility and Quickness

Agility is typically defined as the ability to explosively brake, change direction, and accelerate again, whereas quickness, as defined by Mel Siff, PhD, in his book *Supertraining*, is the ability of the central nervous system to stimulate muscle function without a preliminary stretch. Dr. Siff states further that quickness is elicited without encountering any significant external resistance and without requiring great strength, power, or energy. Although he mentions the central nervous system as the generator of quickness, Dr. Siff acknowledges later in his book that nerve conduction velocities alone do not account for the length and variability of the times measured for quickness in scientific experiments. How can the qualities of quickness and agility be accounted for in the musculoskeletal body?

Refer back to chapter 2, where we discuss the nature of fascia. Visualize having a very intelligent, tactilely sensitive, cooperative, and integrated body stocking beneath your skin that surrounds all your muscles, tendons, ligaments, and bones. Perhaps think of your literal skin as being like a diver's wetsuit, with your fascia being like the skin inside the wetsuit. Try to visualize deeper and see the fascia surrounding and connecting each muscle, organ, and blood vessel. Now, imagine that you see a bug about to fly in your eye and your entire body of fascia, not just the involved eye, reacts by recruiting nearly every single one of your muscles simultaneously to avoid the mishap. Or imagine quickly ducking to avoid getting hit by a baseball coming at you at 95 miles (153 km) per hour. Or think of how hockey players instantly adjust the fine positions of their skates to negotiate high speeds on the ice. This instant messaging to all systems of the body is much faster than a nerve signal, as Dr. Siff indicates. This is because our unrestricted fascial systems function like structures with tensegrity, responding appropriately to any and all movement throughout the body no matter how small or great. Quickness and agility, as well as strength, power, and speed, are highly dependent on an intact and balanced fascial network. These abilities will be compromised if you permit restrictions to freedom of movement to occur. Maintaining flexibility in your fascial body can prevent such restrictions.

At the third level of the performance pyramid, athletes must develop functional skill in their particular sport. As author Gray Cook says in *Athletic Body in Balance* regarding this third level, "A battery of tests assesses ability to do a given activity, participate in a specific sport, or play a specific position within that sport. This level also looks at competition statistics and any specific testing relative to one's sport." To achieve excellence in sport-specific skills and employ them with quickness and agility, you need to be able to generate power on a mobile yet stable base. When all these parts of the performance pyramid are in place, the athlete's only concerns are to maintain mental focus and to keep dynamically relaxed, ready to move when the moment is just right. As athletes participate in practice and get intense coaching at this high level of training to master their skills, they are at increased risk for overtraining, especially after years of training to try to get to this level. For the rest of their careers, they will always be working around their threshold for tolerating high levels of training, always pushing their physical and mental limits to find out what they can really do. Serious nonprofessional but competitive athletes are in a similar situation. Whether you are a professional or nonprofessional, collegiate or high school athlete, you will most likely have athletic trainers, physical therapists, and physicians at your disposal who will help you recover from overtraining and other injuries. It is not our aim in this book to substitute for those practitioners who are dedicated to helping athletes in their respective branch of sports medicine, but to supplement the athlete's "toolbag" of things they can do for themselves to reach a high level of function and skill in sports and athletics. In the next chapter we present a tool called the personal flexibility assessment. It is guaranteed to make you more independent and effective at creating your own stretching program.

chapter 4

Personal Flexibility Assessment

A s you've already learned from the previous chapters, it is not in any athlete's best interest to engage in a stretching program without first evaluating what needs to be stretched. Without an assessment, at best, you may get lucky and experience improved athletic performance from increased flexibility. At worst, you may stretch a part of your body that is already hypermobile and irritate the area by making it too flexible. You can avoid this gamble by creating your personal flexibility assessment (PFA). In doing so, you will learn how to take your personal history, perform a postural evaluation, identify trigger points and create a body map of them, test your range of motion, and test your functional movement patterns. This process will help you clarify any doubts or questions you have about your flexibility, such as why you seem to get tight or sore in the same places. The PFA has been instrumental in helping our clients better understand the causes and effects of their flexibility limitations. This assessment also serves as a personal training record that you can use to reevaluate your progress from time to time.

We've designed the PFA for the healthy, currently uninjured athlete. If you fall outside this category, then we recommend that you seek appropriate guidance from a health professional so that you can get a safe and accurate evaluation and plan for treatment. Once your injury has been stabilized and treated and you are medically cleared, using the PFA on your own is appropriate and will help prevent problems in the future. While we typically conduct a flexibility specialist assessment for our clients in our facility, for the purpose of this book we have modified it and created the PFA for use by individuals.

The PFA is a fundamental element of the Stretch to Win system of individualized flexibility training. Once your assessment is complete, in the following chapters you can learn key stretches and how to build a stretching routine, how to connect the key stretches to the fascial line, and how to reassess and adjust your program for your sport-specific needs and as your flexibility changes. In this chapter we focus on mastering the PFA.

Before you begin your self-assessment, make several photocopies of the PFA form at the end of this chapter, pages 76 to 80, or download a copy from our Web site at www.stretchtowin.com. Use your copies of the self-assessment to write down your findings and answers to the questions. In the future, you can use these as a reference for checking your progress weekly, monthly, or at whatever frequency works with your schedule and goals, and for modifying your program as needed.

In chapter 5 (pages 84 to 94) are two sample completed assessments to help you see how to record the information. Take a moment now to glance over these examples so that when you complete your own assessment, you'll be able to use the symbols and notations that simplify the process.

The PFA has seven steps:

1. Take a brief personal history.
2. Describe any symptoms you are experiencing.
3. Perform a postural evaluation.
4. Test sport-specific movements.
5. Assess your active range of motion (AROM).
6. Identify and map your body's trigger points.
7. Review your findings and look for patterns and correlations.

Step 1: Take a Personal History

The purpose of taking a brief personal history is to review in black and white what events or injuries in your past and present may be contributing to your current condition.

Write down in the personal history section whether you have had any surgeries in the past. No matter what kind of surgery it was, note on your PFA the date of each surgery and on what part of the body it was done. If the surgery was a success and corrected the problem 100 percent, list that separately from those surgeries that did not correct the problem and as a result of which you still experience pain or other symptoms. If there are many, number them chronologically, starting with the most recent episode.

Describe briefly in the current health section any problems, complaints, injuries you have as well as any diagnoses made by a health professional.

Step 2: Describe Your Symptoms

Inflexibility in a healthy, uninjured athlete may be caused by tightness in one or many muscle regions or by stiffness in one or more joints. It may also be reflected in pain and soreness when you do a particular movement. Sometimes you can pinpoint exactly where the tightness, stiffness, or pain is coming from without any problem; at other times the location is more vague, connecting several joints, muscles, tendons, and ligaments.

Record any symptoms you are experiencing by answering the following questions.

1. Do you have any pain or stiffness?* If yes, is the feeling of stiffness or tightness distributed throughout your whole body or is it localized to one area? Start by listing all your symptoms of tightness, stiffness, or pain. Then assign a number to each, with number one being the most tight or sore affected area, number two being the next most affected area, and so on. Once you have completed and ordered your list, using a pencil write the number in a circle on the corresponding area of the body diagram. The number in the circle will represent local pain right in that spot. If you have pain that extends up, down, or around, draw a line and arrow to show in which direction and how far the discomfort extends. Creating an accurate visual record of the location of your discomfort not only allows you to see where you need to focus your work, but it is also an invaluable way to track your progress as you gain flexibility.

   (*If you are in obvious pain or were recently injured, you should seek the help of a health professional before continuing with this profile or a stretching program. If you are sore or in discomfort before, during, or after athletic activity because of stiffness or tightness, continue with this evaluation.)

2. Are there other things that you feel are not quite right with your body, but that you would not describe as pain, stiffness, or tightness? For instance, you may feel or know for a fact that one leg is shorter than the other. This may make you feel uneven or asymmetrical when you walk or run. Another example would be one foot feeling different from the other when you run—its arch may feel collapsed compared to the other foot, or it may feel less stable than the other and be more prone to ankle sprains. Note these observations on the PFA template as part of your numbered list of symptoms and also in the form of a brief comment about exactly what it feels like and how it may be affecting your athletic performance.

Step 3: Perform a Postural Evaluation

Now's the time to get even more honest with yourself by stripping down to your underwear and looking into a full-length mirror. As you'll recall, in chapter 2 we discuss the function of fascia and how patterns of stress and strain are reflected in your posture. The fascia behaves like a net or web, and stress and strain create forces of compression and tension that pull the web out of alignment. When this happens, athletic performance suffers. For example, tightness on one side of the back can disrupt a pitcher's throw, a diver's routine, a gymnast's move, or a basketball player's ability to shoot the ball. This happens because asymmetric tightness interrupts the normal activation patterns of muscles, resulting in less-efficient movement compensations. Compensatory movement patterns eventually cause chronic pain syndromes, which jeopardize athletes' long-term participation in their sport.

Posture assessment is a window through which you can see what areas of the fascia have been pushed or pulled out of alignment. When you correlate the marks you made on the body diagram representing your symptoms with your posture assessment and then compare this with what you feel and see in the following movement and trigger point sections of your PFA, you will be able at last to reach informed conclusions about your flexibility needs. You can then use the findings and conclusions from this continuously updated record to create an individualized flexibility program and modify it as your condition and requirements change. The end result is injury prevention and optimal performance through rapid and accurate problem solving. As you practice using your PFA, you will gain confidence and a measure of personal control over the management of your body and mind. In the process, you'll become more aware and self-reliant as well as healthy.

When you examine your posture in the mirror and look for asymmetries in alignment—differences between the right and left sides, between the front and back, and between the top, middle, and bottom thirds of the body—you are not comparing your body to some concept of perfect alignment of all body regions. Rather, you are looking for a relative symmetry of parts to the whole of the body and a look (and feeling) of length and space in the body. This look and feeling of length and space rather than of compression defines a healthy body that is more fluid than solid (remember that the body is over two-thirds water) and highly mobile. So, when you are observing your body's posture, don't focus on the tiny details—instead, focus on what may seem to you to be obvious differences between one part and another part. The more you practice this kind of observation, the better you'll get at spotting postural imbalances.

This book focuses on stretching the myofascial system for optimal flexibility of your entire body, so we zero in on ways to identify and eliminate restrictions in your myofascia. If the cause of your postural or movement asymmetry lies in your myofascia, then we will be able to help you correct the problem. If our system does not correct the problem, you should see your physician for referral to a practitioner who can give you a proper evaluation. Or, if after working with your PFA for about four weeks you get the impression that the problems you are having are due to poor posture or you cannot seem to move efficiently, consider scheduling an appointment with a specialist in structural integration (see www.theiasi.org to find one), who has unique education and training in changing recalcitrant myofascial structure.

If, like most people, you have a flat full-length mirror that shows only one view of the body at a time (unlike the panoramic-view mirrors you find in fitting rooms), you will focus primarily on the front view of your body. However, when you do use the front view in your PFA, keep in mind the three-dimensional shape of your body, and do your best to mark the other views on the body chart to correlate with what you can see. So, for example, if your right shoulder is lower than the left, mark all views of your PFA—sides and back as well as the front—to show a lower right shoulder.

To help you understand how to assess your own posture, refer to the two sample copies of completed body diagrams depicting clients' self-assessments (see pages 84 to 94). You can adapt and use the symbols shown on these examples to develop your own way of recording what you see and feel when studying your own posture as you complete your assessment on the following areas of the body.

Head

Is your chin in line with the notch at the bottom of your neck, or is it rotated to one side? Does one ear appear lower than the other, showing that your head is slightly tilted? Mark down any asymmetries and misalignments you can see. These signs, among others, may be due to tightness in joint, ligament, or myofascial structures. One reason why your head position is important is that your eyes will rotate in their sockets to accommodate any asymmetry. This often happens after whiplash and other head and neck injuries. It may also come from a poor habitual posture, like many people assume when they work in front of a computer terminal all day; these individuals start slumping their spines and craning their heads forward as they sit all day, peering into the screen. This forward head position creates shear forces in the neck, with the lower part of the neck flexing too much while the upper part of the neck hyperextends too much. We call this having a "turtle head" position, and it eventually creates a compensatory rotation of the eyes in the socket such that they turn downward, looking down the nose. There are many reflexive movements initiated with the eyes that directly activate muscles throughout your body; any change in eye and head position will have a trickle-down effect on the rest of the body. This trickle-down effect will create additional compensations during athletic movement and eventual problems from the extra stress and strain on your myofascial system.

An example of a different trickle-down effect is shown by a right-handed golfer whose head is slightly rotated to the right of center. Her eyes naturally counter this head rotation to the right with a compensatory rotation left. When she drives the ball, she will have to make other adjustments in her body to deal with the fact that her head cannot keep a left-rotated position relative to the rest of her body during the backswing. In fact, she might have a chronic inability to get into her ideal position when she drives a ball, with the result that she forces her swing instead of flowing with it. When an experienced athlete forces a movement instead of flowing with it, we consider this a cardinal sign of a flexibility deficit. We have seen this confirmed many times in our clinic.

Shoulders

Are the collarbones horizontal and lined up with each other, or does one or both angle upward or downward? Is the point of one shoulder higher or lower than the corresponding point on the other? Does one shoulder appear to be shifted more forward than the other? Mark any differences you see.

One statistic states that, viewed from the front, approximately 85 percent of right-handed people's right shoulders are lower than their left shoulders. Various professionals debate whether to consider this a normal state, since so many people have this discrepancy without any apparent problems or pain.

Of course, there is no perfect or ideal posture. How could there be with the variety of human shapes on this earth? Still, we do find it helpful to observe whether one shoulder is tighter or more compressed or significantly not in line with the other side. Any discrepancy you see statically will be confirmed dynamically when you start moving the problem side later in this assessment.

What we commonly see in the clinic is that the shoulder of an athlete's dominant arm is not only lower but also pulled more forward than the less-dominant side. The significance of this is that a forward shoulder can start to literally drag or pull on structures in the neck. This can lead to a compensated neck position that in turn may create a pinched nerve or disc bulges. Hopefully you can see that it's better to prevent this kind of problem before it becomes a permanent injury.

Ribs

Does the rib cage as a whole appear centered, or is it shifted to the left or right? Is one side of the rib cage more prominent, sticking out more to the front? The effects of a rib cage that is shifted or rotated more to one side are similar to those of an asymmetrical head position. When you need to perform an athletic movement that requires your rib cage to move freely to the opposite side of the deviation, such as swinging a bat or racket, you will encounter some form of resistance to the movement in your body. You will have to either force the movement, which is inefficient and ultimately injurious to your body, or perform a compensated movement, a "detour" path of swing when you move that bat or racket. Over time, you may get good at adapting your swing or other movement, but it will come at the cost of eventually stressing or straining your body. Medications only mask the cumulative damage that is growing each time you move this way.

Pelvis

With the palms facing the floor and the fingers pointing straight ahead, press the edges of the hands to the upper sides of the pelvis. Is one side higher than the other? If one side of the pelvis is higher than the other, this may indicate that the leg on that side is longer, which obviously means that the other leg is shorter, not in the bone but owing to some myofascial tightness in your body. One common contributor to this situation is the quadratus lumborum (QL) muscle, which is a deep back and waist muscle that connects your lower ribs to the top of your pelvis and both of those areas to almost every bone in your lumbar spine. Another muscle that may functionally shorten your leg if it is tight, is a deep one called the psoas. This rather long muscle is part of what controls your posture, and it connects to every bone in your lower spine then travels across your hip joint to attach to the inside of your femur or thigh bone. Legs of uneven length can cause problems running, skating, jumping, or performing any sport that works the legs. Neck, shoulder, back, hip, knee, ankle, and foot pain or dysfunction in movement can all result from a functionally short leg. Once you've identified the contributors to this problem, you can make a plan to fix it.

Hips

You can quickly learn a great deal about the flexibility of your hips by looking at your knee and foot position as you view it in the mirror. We address those areas in detail later in the assessment, but here we will discuss their relevance to your hips.

What we commonly see with tight hips is that the knee and foot on one or both sides is turned outward. In what is considered a normal and relaxed position for the feet the toes may point out slightly, but the kneecaps generally still point straight ahead. With a tighter-than-normal hip, the knee and foot will face significantly outward compared to the normal position just described. Consequently, walking, running, and lunging movements are less efficient, decreasing speed and power and increasing the chance for injury. Note your own kneecap and foot positions so that you can see if they correlate with tightness in your deep hip external rotators, the layer of muscles lying beneath the large gluteus maximus.

Knees

Look at your kneecaps. If your feet are placed directly under your hips and comfortably toed out slightly, do your kneecaps point straight ahead, as they generally should, or is one or both rotated inward or outward? Are both knees bowed in, perhaps even touching each other (genu valgus), or are they bowed out (genu varum), or is just one knee affected? Are both or one knee hyperextended (genu recurvatum) or are both or one slightly flexed? Mark which way your knees are pointing on your PFA.

The position, or placement, of your knees depends partly on what you were born with, partly on the shape and function of your hips and the arches of your feet, and partly on the position of your feet in a given moment. When a knee has to function with a suboptimal alignment, whatever the cause, it becomes more susceptible to injury. The ligaments that stabilize knees are vulnerable to sprains and ruptures when they have to function under the repetitive strain conditions that misalignment can create. For example, the anterior cruciate ligament may have a complete rupture after an athlete does a move he or she has done safely many times in the past.

Feet

Look down and see if you stand with the feet relatively parallel or slightly toed out to each other. If their angles are quite different from each other or greatly toed out or in, recheck them by marching in place for a few steps, stopping, and then looking again to see if there is a change. If your feet place differently after the march, your original standing position was probably a little out of balance. If the placement is the same after the march, you can consider it a reliable indicator of how you stand. Does one foot or both feet point in or out from the parallel? If you look at them in the mirror, do you find that one or both arches collapse, that is, they seem pretty flat to the ground; or are they high enough to make you bear more weight on the outside of the foot?

The way you naturally place your feet is a good indicator of what kinds of stress and strain the knees and hips are under. If your arches are too low or touch the floor (pronated feet) and they still give you problems after trying our system, then getting orthotics from a recommended practitioner such as a podiatrist may be in order. If you are in the minority and have the opposite problem of high arches (supinated feet), you should also see a specialist who can advise you on proper athletic footwear. In either case, getting your feet—the literal foundation of your body—functioning correctly will automatically improve the structural balance and function of the rest of your body.

Finally, close your eyes and get a sense of how you stand. Does your stance feel evenly distributed onto both feet or do you feel that you bear more weight on one side? Maybe more weight is exerted on the heels or balls of the feet (or perhaps you feel this in one foot only). When you have a good sense of the way you stand, mentally scan your body from head to toe and note any areas of tension, tightness, or soreness. Record these on your PFA, describing what you feel in words and marking where you feel it on the figure diagram. This is a great starting point from which to begin to track the way your body looks, feels, and performs.

Step 4: Test Sport-Specific Movements

In this part of the PFA, you will assume several body positions that are common to your sport and that serve as good indicators of how flexible you are. To perform at your best in your sport, the act of getting into and out of these positions should be smooth and free of any problems or symptoms. Try each position change at slow and fast speeds. There should be a feeling of strength and stability. Depending on your sport, try moving into and out of multiple positions in various directions. You should also perform a few dynamic sport movements, such as an explosive start for a sprint or a cutting move to each side. Try some advanced combinations, varying the speed and direction of movement. Note on your PFA any tightness, discomfort, or lack of flow anywhere in your body. You will use this test again later to check the effect that performing self-myofascial release (sMFR) and stretching has on the movements.

Step 5:
Assess Your Active Range of Motion

Now that you have put down on paper your physical history and symptoms, examined your posture, and sport-specific movements, it is time to look at some simple movement patterns and how you perform them in order to assess your overall active range of motion (AROM). If you perform simple movements incorrectly because you have inadequate range of motion to do them properly, or if they are painful, then complex movements with added forces like those encountered in sports and fitness training will be problematic. For example, if the AROM of someone who is training to be a baseball pitcher has shoulder movements deficient in external rotation and abduction, then that pitcher will sooner or later develop severe problems not only in his shoulder but also in the rest of his body due to the compensations that must occur. Even if you don't detect any imbalances during your first assessment, it's a good idea to check again from time to time to see if you've remained in balance after a hard day's workout, game, or competition.

The AROM assessment offers a simple, logical, and quick way to get a good picture of your general flexibility at any given point in time. The assessment that we use is familiar to doctors, therapists, and trainers, so athletes who learn how to assess their own AROM with it will be better able to communicate with their medical and other support staff as well.

Before starting, it is essential to keep in mind that, as with posture, there is no such thing as ideal flexibility. But we do need to have some kind of reference for what is "normal" when we move. What has worked exceptionally well for us is to tell our clients that normal movement feels pain free and effortless.

Pain free needs no explanation; *effortless* means that your movements are easy and smooth. You should not be holding your breath when you do any of the movements in this assessment; if you catch yourself doing so, you will need to determine whether there is some restriction that is making you hold your breath. Smooth movement flows without any evidence of tension, shaking, or popping or cracking sounds. Many of us get so used to ignoring these signs from our bodies that our movements are not optimal. The problem is compounded when, after years of our ignoring these signs of structural imbalance, they develop into more serious and chronic problems such as tendinitis, bursitis, and osteo-arthritis. All these problems tend to afflict professional athletes at earlier ages than the general public.

What is considered "optimal" flexibility is often contingent upon a given sport's movement requirements. For some sports it might even be beneficial to have certain areas of excessive flexibility that would normally be considered det-rimental when found in this kind of assessment. For instance, it is advantageous for breaststroke swimmers to have excessive flexibility (or hypermobility) in their knees, for their most effective kick. On the other hand, while this flexibility might serve them well in the pool, if they do not also work on maintaining good stability in the knees they can develop severe problems that will progressively deteriorate the joints, forcing them to quit swimming and to deal with lifelong knee problems. The point is that you must gain the flexibility appropriate to your activity, no more and no less. Candid discussions with your coach and trainer about what is specifically needed for your sport will help you to determine this. Then, with your completed PFA, you will be able to identify many potential sources of flexibility problems before they become serious.

General Spine Movements

We begin this assessment with the spine because it is the literal center of the body and it contains the spinal cord, a part of your central nervous system. Your brain and spinal cord are covered with several layers of connective tissue that is prone to getting restricted in its flexibility, just like any other region of fascia. For instance, one reason some people who get a whiplash injury never seem to get completely better is that they develop restrictions to normal movement in the fascia that covers the brain and spinal cord. This fascia also commonly gets tight from mental and physical stress and strain. When this happens, some people feel generalized, deep tightness in all their muscles, while others get a specific area of tightness, such as in the neck or back. Naturally, you will not be able to perform at your best in this kind of scenario.

1. Stand in front of a mirror with your feet hip-width apart.
2. Bend forward at the waist, keeping the knees straight but not locked. By just letting go and not forcing the movement you will naturally stop moving at a point where the slack of the soft tissues along the back of the legs, hips, pelvis, and trunk has been completely taken up without any extra exertion to get more range of motion (figure 4.1a).
3. Mark on the chart where the middle fingers touch the leg or the floor. Note whether one hand reaches farther than the other, which could mean that you have a hypermobile shoulder on the longer-reaching side or a hypomobile shoulder on the opposite side. Note whether one hand seems to reach more outside the knee while the other is more inside the knee.

This may be because you are tilting out from the trunk in the direction of the outside hand, possibly indicating tightness in the trunk or waist on the side you are tilting toward. Also note what areas in your body most seem to limit the motion and what parts feel the tightest. Common restrictions to this movement and places where many may feel tight are in the low back, glutes, hamstrings, and calf muscles. Exceptionally tight people will also feel it in the mid to upper back and neck.

4. Return to standing upright and place the palms, with the fingers pointing down toward the heels, on the very top of your buttocks where they meet the back of the pelvis and low back. Slowly bend the spine backward, keeping the knees as straight as possible but allowing the pelvis to glide slightly forward so that you don't feel

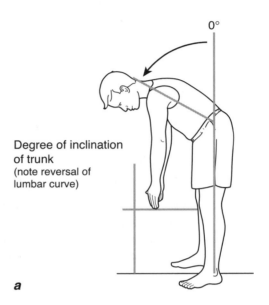

Degree of inclination
of trunk
(note reversal of
lumbar curve)

a

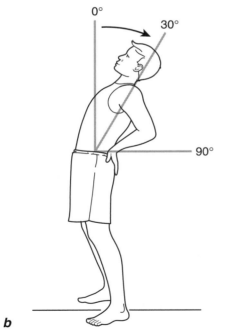

b

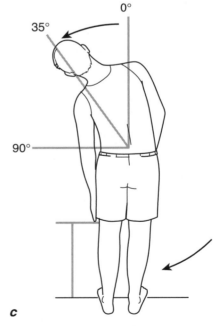

c

Figure 4.1   General spine assessments: forward flexion *(a)*; extension *(b)*; and lateral flexion *(c)*.

as if you are about to lose your balance (figure 4.1*b*). Notice whether the center or sides of your low back feel tighter or more compressed, and notice any area where you feel inflexible or where you feel a block to the movement. People who are very tight in the hips may feel it in the front of the hips and into the lower abdomen on one or both sides, where the psoas muscle is buried deeply on either side of your spine. Return to the upright position and indicate on the body chart wherever you feel symptoms.

5. Now lean over to one side, bending at the waist, and then to the other side, letting the arms hang naturally at your sides. Note any difference between the two sides and whether you feel it in the neck, ribs, waist, hips, back, or other part of the body. Also note where your hand touches your leg and whether or not this is the same on the opposite side (figure 4.1*c*).

Upper Extremity General Movements

If you do not have any obvious problems with the neck, arms, and shoulders, look carefully for differences in the look and feel of the movements that you perform. Tightness in the neck or in the muscles between the neck and shoulder (such as the upper trapezius) may cause one or both shoulders to "hunch" when you raise your arms overhead. The possible implications of this situation are many; among them, you may be more prone to getting a pinched nerve in the neck and you may not flow as well with movements like throwing a ball or swimming. You can check the main upper extremity movements by using the following procedure:

1. Stand in front of a full-length mirror with the feet hip-width apart, making sure that you have a good view of your shoulders and hips when you move them. You might make some big circles with your arms to see how far back you need to stand in order to see most or all of them.

   Return your arms to the starting position straight down by the sides. Now, facing the mirror straight on, move the arms straight behind you, bending the elbows slightly. Compare and contrast hand and arm position for asymmetries. This is called shoulder extension (shown in figure 4.2*a*). To get a truer reading, try to keep the rest of your body erect, resisting the tendency to tilt your trunk forward to get the arms up higher. As you did when you viewed your shoulder flexion from the side, turn 90 degrees from the mirror so you can see how far the arm goes up from the side. Compare sides, recording any differences on your PFA.

2. Slowly raise both arms straight up in front of you until they are fully overhead and your shoulders are as high up as they can go. This is called shoulder flexion (figure 4.2*a*). Now do this with just your left arm in a different view—turn away from the mirror 90 degrees to the right so that

you have to turn your head left to see how high you can lift the arm. Then face the opposite direction and repeat with the right arm, looking for differences between the sides. Note both the angle where your range stops and the reason it stops there—is it painful, or does it just stop because that is the limit of its movement? Normal flexion of the shoulder is about 180 degrees (with "zero" meaning the arm is straight down by the leg), so that viewed from the side, when your arm is completely over-head it should be aligned with your leg. Estimate each arm's range of motion using the guide in the figure draw-ing, and note how the shoul-der and upper arm feel while doing the movement and at the end of the movement.

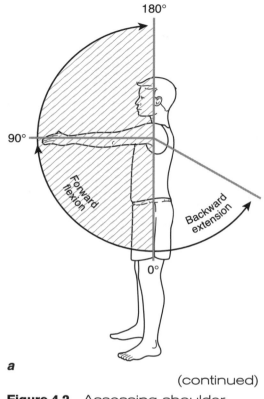

(continued)

Figure 4.2 Assessing shoulder flexion and extension.

3. Now, keeping your arms straight, move them outward and upward from your sides in what is called abduction (figure 4.2*b*). Normal abduction movement is 180 degrees. This is similar to flexion, except the path of movement to get to the same endpoint is different, requiring different patterns of muscle, tendon, ligament, and fascia use. Again, note your range of motion for each arm and any tightness, pain, or blocks to move-ment on your PFA. Restrictions in this movement typically involve your rotator cuff and other muscles of the shoulder that stabilize your humerus (upper arm bone) during simple movements. Any lack of smoothness in this movement indicates either a lack of proper motor control or a lack of proper ligament and tendon stability. While the former can be managed through working with our system, if you suspect the latter (experienced as disturbing clicks, clunks, or unchanging pain when moving the shoulder or arm) you may need to see an orthopedist to rule out serious injury before you undertake the stretches in this system. Either scenario will create problems for athletes, especially those who use their arm to throw or shoot balls.

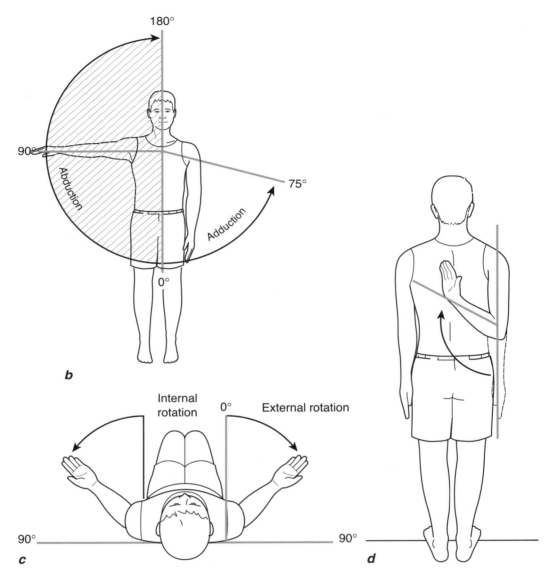

Figure 4.2 Assessing other body movements: abduction and adduction *(b)*; internal and external rotation *(c)*; reaching behind the back *(d)*.

4. Return again to the starting position. Next, with your palms facing forward, bend at the elbows and raise just the forearms until the elbows are flexed to 90 degrees (a right angle) from the straight-down position (figure 4.2*c*). Now move the hands outward, keeping the elbows immobile by your sides. Start with the thumbs pointing away from the center of the body so that they point outward and then more backward until movement stops. Note any difference in comfort and range of motion between the two arms on your PFA. Normal ROM is about 80 to 90 degrees from the start-

ing position right in front of you. Without going into the biomechanical details, you need full flexibility here if you are to lift your shoulders and arms overhead without strain. For example, if you do weightlifting with inflexible shoulders you are asking for lots of shoulder problems down the road.

5. Finally, turn around so that you can see your back in the mirror. Reach one arm and hand up behind the back, with the hand aiming for the area between the shoulder blades. Note where your thumb touches your back on your PFA (figure 4.2*d*). Repeat on the other side, noting how your shoulder feels and the location and amount of any difference in the range of motion. Wrestlers and others may need this motion more than some other athletes. Still, all athletes need to have excellent mobility in every direction that the joints move, especially the ones that are used in their sport. This mobility will help prevent the early degenerative changes in joints, like osteoarthritis and disc disease, that are so common in sports. Maintaining this mobility by periodically doing the PFA and following the indications drawn from it will lengthen your participation in sports and keep your body healthier in the process.

Using the results of your PFA and periodically reevaluating your flexibility with it will allow you to focus on stretching the areas that you have found to help your function. But you will also find yourself periodically taking more time, maybe in the off-season or on some weekends, to get the full benefits of more generalized stretching to increase your overall flexibility and mobility.

Lower Extremity General Movements

These movements are especially important to assess for most sports because most sports require optimal hip flexibility. But most any activity can benefit from increased range of motion in the lower extremity.

1. Stand in front of the mirror and raise one knee straight up in front of you, bending the leg. Note how high the top of the knee goes and how it feels in your hip and in the rest of the body. Also note whether you can do this movement freely from the hip joint only or must bend the standing knee or your trunk toward the lifted knee. Then do the same with the other knee and compare with the height and feeling of the first. Record the results on your PFA. This movement, which is called hip flexion (figure 4.3), is extremely important in enabling you to perform a wide variety of functional patterns. While rock climbers, gymnasts, and martial artists who do high kicks may need more of this ROM, the inability to do this movement and feel that it is light, easy, and effortless indicates some underlying problems that will cause trouble for many athletes, such as tightness in the deep muscles around the hip joint. The body is wired so that when you move through a range of motion, the muscles that would oppose

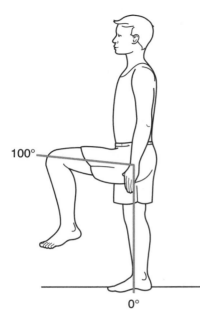

100°

0°

Figure 4.3 Assessing hip flexion.

that motion, usually called antagonists, let go, thus permitting the movement to occur. In this case, if the glutes or one of the deeper muscles in the back of the hip such as the piriformis have a trigger point, the muscle may contract when you are trying to flex the hip. You'll still be able to do it, but it will likely feel heavier or less smooth than the other hip. If you have this problem in sports, when you perform a movement such as running a football or soccer ball, you will use even more muscular effort to do so. This inefficient way of moving has a trickle-down (and trickle–up) effect that can make the knee joint less stable and more vulnerable to injury. Guess which joint is one of the most commonly injured in sports!

With this movement you are also assessing the standing leg's ability to remain straight, which is called hip extension, while the other hip is flexing. The standing leg has to have adequate flexibility in its hip flexors and groin muscles (called hip adductors) to allow the other leg to be pulled up and away from its neighbor. When they are tight, you will compensate by bending the standing knee and overflexing the spine in order to get the other knee up. This compensation leaves the back and knee in a less stable and more vulnerable position, thus increasing the risk of further injury. Even if you do not do high kicks for your sport as American football punters do, assessing hip flexion gives you a reference for your progress in your overall flexibility.

2. Repeat the previous instruction with the first leg, but when you reach the end of the movement take both hands and clasp them around your knee to see how much higher it can go and how your body feels when you do this. Does the assisted leg move easily, or is there resistance? Assisting the movement with your hands focuses the movement more on the hip joint because the muscles around it are more relaxed with your help. Again, repeat with the other leg and note any differences on your PFA. One common symptom is a pinching sensation in the front of your hip, right in the crease that is made with this motion. This usually indicates tightness in the front of the hip fascia or in the deep hip flexor tendon of the iliacus and psoas muscles. This problem is most common for athletes who explode powerfully in running or jumping sports. Yet it can also often be found in people who sit for much of the day, thereby effectively locking up their hip capsule and flexor tendons that cross in front of the joint.

Spine Combination Movement

While the above movements give you some useful information about the way you function, they do not provide as complete a picture as combination movements in which several body parts move simultaneously in familiar patterns. These combination movements can give you a rough idea of how you might feel and function with real everyday movements and are thus a reliable benchmark of how your flexibility program is working. Combination movements also can serve as a helpful gauge of how you respond to treatment. In order to keep your PFA as concise and helpful as possible for self-assessment, we have condensed the longer version we use in our clinic into the following brief version.

1. Stand with your back to a clock or other object that is at eye height. Look over one shoulder by turning the head, the neck, the chest, and so on down your body, section by section, until you take up all the slack all the way down to the ankles. Note on your PFA where the movement feels most blocked or least free. Repeat the movement from the other side and record these results. Is the restriction higher or lower on one side than the other, for example? Can you see the object better or see farther past it from one side than from the other? Naturally, if you can turn around farther on one side than the other, you might think that you need to stretch the restricted side. But if the more mobile side hurt when you were twisting, it may be because you have a spinal segment that moved more than its fair share. This is a form of hypermobility. On account of the pain, the hypermobile side is the problem side in this case, not the less-mobile, pain-free side. The task is to find which areas of the spine are not moving enough during the combination movement, thereby forcing the hypermobile area to move more in compensation. While only a qualified manual therapist or chiropractor is adept at identifying and treating individual vertebral segments that are not moving correctly, you will be able to identify tight or stiff areas above and below the painful hypermobile areas so that later you can release them through self-myofascial release (see chapter 5) and through the stretching techniques we show beginning in chapter 6. If you have no pain but do feel distinctly different moving one side compared to the other, such as moving with more ease, then there may be an error in muscles that are supposed to move in sequence. Many times, you can alleviate this by treating the areas where you've found trigger points in the course of these assessments. They may also be alleviated by stretching the muscles that you have found are inhibiting the movements in these assessments.

2. Now place your feet shoulder-width apart and bend your knees deeply but without letting your heels come up from the floor. Repeat the movement of the previous instruction on each side. If you feel the rotation differently or more intensely in the hips, back, or pelvis, note this on your PFA, along with any differences between sides.

Upper Extremity Combination Movement

Again, assessing this movement is crucial for the athlete who does a lot of overhead motions but important as well for everyone who wants a healthy shoulder.

1. Stand in front of the mirror with the hands by your sides and palms resting on the sides of your thighs. Bend the elbows so that the fingers point out and the palms face each other in front. Now, maintaining the 90-degree bend at the elbow, raise the elbows out to the sides until they are in line with the shoulders, forming a 90-degree angle with the trunk. (This position is also referred to as "elbows flexed 90 degrees and shoulders abducted 90 degrees.")

2. Maintaining this angle between the upper arm and body, lift the hands upward and backward so that the fingers now point straight up to the ceiling (also known as externally rotating the shoulders 90 degrees, see figure 4.2c). Note any differences between sides in range of motion and any restriction or pain on your PFA, as well as any changes in your posture that occur. For example, many athletes who have restrictions or other problems in the ROM of one shoulder tend to raise it more toward the ear than the other shoulder during this test. Be sure to note such symptoms on your PFA , as they can be especially problematic for athletes who throw or swim, but it is important for everyone to optimize this area.

3. Rotate the forearms and hands back down so the palms are once again parallel to and facing the floor and try to rotate the hands further, palms facing behind you into what is called internal rotation (see figure 4.2c). When you do this, try to keep the elbows up, but without tensing the neck and shoulders up to the ears. If you are unable to do this, your joint capsule or your rotator cuff is very tight in this direction; if you have significant pain, clicks, clunks, or a feeling of giving way in either direction, some structure may be torn, in which case you need to see a shoulder orthopedist. View both of these ranges from the side, as you did before. You might also want to check how they move in opposite directions simultaneously, looking for smoothness of movement and flawless coordination. Record the results on your PFA.

4. Now combine steps 2 and 3 above, rotating one arm externally and the other internally. Reverse, and then note any differences or symptoms.

Lower Extremity Combination Movement

While you may think this test is not essential if you don't do squats in the weight room, think of all the variations of the motions that you've done or seen in sports: football stance, sprinters block position, baseball field ready position, volleyball or tennis ready position, and so on. Many athletic positions have modified two-

and one-leg squats of some type, so this motion test is very helpful for picking out asymmetries and other problems.

1. Stand in front of the mirror with the feet slightly wider than the hips. Squat as far down as you can easily balance, looking for any of the following errors in movement: feet starting to turn outward (possible tight peroneals); knees turning outward (possible tight hip external rotators); or back rounding excessively, with the trunk leaning forward (possible tight hip flexors or deep hip external rotators). Mark any of these on your PFA.

2. Now step back 6 to 8 feet (1.8 to 2.4 m) from the mirror so that you have room to lunge. Begin by standing with the feet hip-width apart. Step out with one foot and lunge forward until the back knee just starts to touch the ground. Your front knee should bend over the center of your foot; it should not pass over the toes. If your knee leans inward, this may be due to tightness in the groin or psoas. If it leans outward, tight hip external rotators could be the cause. If the back, hip, or thigh feels like it restricts the movement, you could have tightness in those regions as well as in the hip flexors or quadriceps. Repeat on the other side and note the results on your PFA.

Step 6: Identify Trigger Points

A trigger point (often described as a knot) is a taut local band of myofascia that is very sensitive but also quite responsive to progressively deeper levels of externally applied pressure. This step in the flexibility assessment will teach you how to identify active trigger points in your own body so that you can eliminate a significant cause of decreased athletic performance. You'll also learn how to identify latent or hidden trigger points so that you can eliminate them with a combination of self-myofascial release (sMFR) and stretching before they start causing problems. This chapter helps you identify problems and imbalances; you will learn how to deal with them in chapter 5.

Please note that several conditions are contraindications to performing this part of the assessment. Do not roll on the balls if you are receiving anticoagulant therapy or suffer from malignancy, osteoporosis, osteomyelitis, acute rheumatoid arthritis, inflammatory conditions, systemic or localized infection, sensitive diabetes, circulatory conditions (e.g., edema, hematoma, blood pressure conditions), open wounds, stitches, fractures, or hypersensitive skin conditions. Also be aware that this can be very powerful and intense work. If you ever feel dizzy, light headed, or nauseated, please stop immediately.

To identify trigger points you will need a minimum of two balls: one racquet ball or tennis ball (or a Footsie Roller, if you have one) and one firm 5-inch (13-cm) diameter rubberized ball that has a little give to it when you press it.

Athletes who are taller than 6 feet (183 cm) or weigh more than 200 pounds (91 kg) may want to also use the 7-inch (18 cm) ball, which can cover more surface area. If you don't have either the 5- or 7-inch balls but do have a firm foam roll, you can use that instead, but we prefer the ball because of its increased specificity, relatively small size, and portability compared to the foam roll. You will use the smaller tennis or racquet ball to find trigger points in the feet and the larger ball (or a foam roll) to find them in the rest of the body. You will also need to find a floor that is firm but also has some resilience, such as an athletic-room floor or a carpeted surface; most people need to get used to the pressure of the ball on their body before they can roll on it over a hard floor.

Figure 4.4, *a* through *e*, shows you the myofascial lines that will guide you as you roll on the ball. Use these illustrations to also guide your markings on your PFA. Mark any areas where you notice tightness and tenderness, as well as the direction of any pain that radiates outward from where you are rolling the ball.

You will start with your feet, which have important acupuncture points that act as gauges for the entire body (the hands and head also have similar points that will not be discussed in this book). This is because the feet are both beginning and terminal points for the acupuncture meridians—channels in your fascia that store, move, and dispel energy, blood, and water throughout your body. We also start with the feet since they are the foundation of your posture and of your movements.

You can see in figure 4.4, *a* through *e*, that the fascial lines begin at the feet, run up the body then down the other side, ending at the feet again. Consequently, assessing (and, later, treating) your feet first can give you a reliable idea not only of what is going on in the feet but also of what is going on in the rest of the body. Since we are not discussing acupuncture in this book, suffice it to say that eliminating any trigger points in the feet can only benefit the rest of the body. And because the feet are the base for just about all functional movement especially in athletics, unblocking restrictions in the feet will help unblock other areas of the body.

1. Place a tennis or racquet ball or a Footsie Roller on a carpeted or athletic-room floor that has some give to it. If you have poor balance, stand facing a wall, counter, or stable piece of furniture that will not move when you lean on it.

2. If you are using a surface as a support, place both hands on it. Place one foot on the ball so that it is under the center of your heel. If you have any heel pain or problems, position the ball just in front of the heel, under the arch, instead.

3. Slowly shift more of your weight onto the ball to increase the pressure under the foot. Stop increasing the pressure the moment you feel discomfort or pain under the ball; get off it and note the location of the discomfort on your PFA. If the discomfort radiates outward, make an arrow that shows where it starts and ends.

4. Get back on the ball and continue in like fashion heading toward your toes, slowly moving your foot over the ball, stepping on it with as much pressure as tolerated and stopping only to note the places where you feel significant discomfort on your PFA. Remember that each time you move the ball forward to a new spot, you begin with light pressure and slowly increase it to see how it feels, then ease off before moving to the next spot.

5. When you are done with one foot, repeat the process on the other. Note that, like any new skill it takes more time to learn it in the beginning; as you make this a regular part of your training, you will assess and effectively treat yourself in seconds to a few minutes.

Now you are ready to find trigger points in the rest of the body using the bigger ball. Before you begin, note that you should not use the ball to put pressure on any of the following areas: the coccyx (tailbone); the lower eleventh and twelfth ribs (the floating ribs), which start in the mid to low back region and extend to your sides above the pelvis; any part of the front of your abdomen, from the bottom tip of your breastbone down to the bottom of the pelvis and out to the sides above your pelvis and below the ribs; the genital area; any part of the neck; or any other areas that are too sensitive to tolerate pressure.

Superficial Back Line

The superficial back line (SBL; figure 4.4a) connects the entire posterior surface of the body from

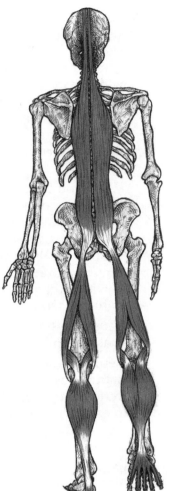

Figure 4.4a The superficial back line (SBL).

Reprinted from *Anatomy trains*, T. Myers, p. 60, 2001, with permission from Elsevier.

the bottom of the foot to the top of the head. When standing, the SBL functions as one continuous line of integrated fascia and frequently reflects symptoms of tightness in the back of the knees, hamstrings, and low back in our clients.

While this line provides a good basic reference for the line you follow for this assessment, the assessment includes some detours and variations. We encourage you to explore and find out for yourself what works best for you.

1. Sit on the floor, leaning back with your legs in front of you and bent at the knees, your feet pointing forward on the floor, and your hands on the floor behind you with the fingers pointing away from you.

2. Position the ball on your sacrum just above the tailbone, and start a very slow roll, moving the upper body just a little, perhaps by leaning to one side and then the other, to better maneuver the ball into the flat bone of your sacrum and your muscles. Roll approximately the distance of the width of the ball in one direction, return to the central position, and then change directions and roll out another width of the ball, still sitting on it. Do this one time very slowly—to the left, to the right, and upward (but not downward, since you don't want to put pressure on the coccyx). If you find a trigger point, note its location and the direction of any radiating discomfort on your PFA.

3. When you have finished rolling out over the sacrum, pick one side and roll farther outward, past the high buttock, to reach your side. You will need to start turning your body to the side in order to roll over all the muscles that attach to the outside hip bone and on up to the outside of the pelvis, called the iliac crest. Review figure 4.4*a* for guidance as to what direction to roll in. This is one of the key regions that restrict low back, pelvis, and hip flexibility. On the PFA, note any areas that are especially tight and tender as well as anywhere the discomfort radiates outward.

4. Return to the sacrum area and repeat instruction 3 on the opposite side, making similar notes of any signs or symptoms.

5. Return to the sacrum area. Now begin to progress up your spinal column, starting just off the side of the spinal bone. Work the muscles around each vertebra, rolling 2 to 3 inches (5 to 8 cm) outward and back before you move up to the next segment. Going slowly, repeat this sequence all the way up the back to the shoulder. Return to the sacrum and repeat on the other side.

6. Roll on the ball between the shoulder blade and the spine. Go as high as you can toward the top before the shoulder rounds too much for you to roll on it accurately. Now go back to the area between your spine and your shoulder blade and slowly roll your body over so the ball is on the blade itself, which is covered by your rotator cuff muscles. Take your time and explore all the regions of the shoulder blade while you are on your back. Stop at this point and do not perform this assessment on the arm and hand as doing so is not as effective without personal instruction. Repeat on the other side.

7. Take another look at figure 4.4*a* and examine the way the line of fascia moves from the pelvis and down the leg. Upon finishing both sides of the back and shoulders, go back down to one buttock, starting at the "sits bone" at the bottom of the buttock, which is what you rest on when you sit in a chair. This is where most of the hamstring muscles originate.

8. Continue slowly down the back of the thigh (the hamstrings), noting any trigger points you find along the way. Then slowly roll the ball down your lower leg, starting just below the knee joint and proceeding down

the calf to finish near the Achilles tendon at the heel. Repeat the sequence on the other side.

Congratulations, you have just finished most of the important areas of the superficial back line of fascia. If this is the first time that you have ever done this, get up and walk around after assessing each side. Even though this is the assessment part and not the treatment part, you cannot help but start to feel a decrease in some of the pressure, tightness, and soreness of the trigger points that you have just rolled over.

Lateral Line

The lateral line (LL, figure 4.4b) traverses each side of the body from the medial and lateral mid-point of the foot around the outside of the ankle and up the lateral aspect of the leg and thigh, passing along the trunk in a basket weave pattern to the skull in the region of the ear. This line of fascia frequently is responsible for creating a functional short leg, contributing to athletic imbalance and unilateral pain.

Even though the lateral line is continuous going up the side of the body, you will avoid rolling over sensitive areas like the ribs. In this assessment you focus on the line as it proceeds from the pelvis to the ankle.

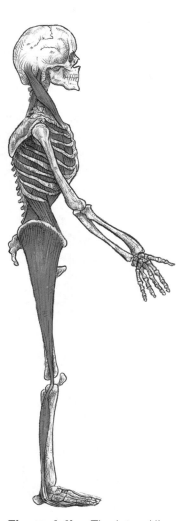

Figure 4.4b   The lateral line (LL).

Reprinted from *Anatomy trains*, T. Myers, p. 120, 2001, with permission from Elsevier.

1. Lie on your side on the floor. Prop yourself up, supporting your upper body on the forearm of the bottom arm and keeping the hand of the top arm on the floor out in front of you.

2. Place the ball under the side of the bottom leg, just above the outside hip bone (known as the greater trochanter of the femur) but below the top of the pelvis. You are now on the large gluteus medius muscle.

3. Place the top leg out in front of you and separate it from the bottom one. Rest the lower part of the top leg with foot and knee on the floor so that, combined with the position of your arms and hands, you have three points of stability for side leg rolling. Explore this fan-shaped region which contains muscles responsible for the balance of your low back, pelvis, hip, knee, and foot when you walk and run. Those muscles also guide the leg

when you move it out to the side and away from your body. Because of all the use this area gets, it is often tender, but it is particularly so as you descend below the hip to the knee.

4. In the same way you went over the other areas, proceed slowly down the side of the leg below the outside bone of the hip (greater trochanter) and slowly start to roll over what is called the iliotibial band (ITB). Note the tightest, most tender areas on your evaluation.

5. When you get to the level of the knee, get your legs in line with your upper body and stack your legs on top of one another, balancing on the hand of the topmost arm, the forearm of your bottom arm, and your bottom hip bone. Skip over the knee joint and slowly begin to roll on the outside calf. The peroneal muscles in this area are usually tender in athletes who pronate their feet. Stop when you can no longer maintain balance over the ball or when you have rolled to just above the ankle bone.

6. Repeat on the opposite side. Get up and walk around to ascertain whether you feel any different in the areas just rolled on compared with the rest of your body.

Superficial Front Line

The superficial front line (SFL, figure 4.4c) connects the entire anterior surface of the body from the top of the feet to the front side of the skull; when the hip is extended, as in standing, it acts as one continuous line of integrated myofascia. Key points along this line get particularly short and tight in people who spend a great deal of the day sitting.

Note that even though the line of fascia traverses the abdomen and ribs, you do not roll over those areas.

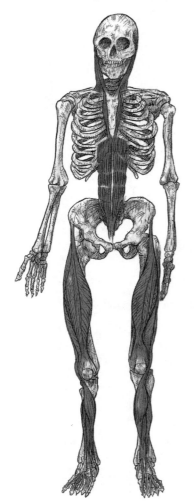

Figure 4.4c The superficial front line (SFL).

Reprinted from *Anatomy trains*, T. Myers, p. 92, 2001, with permission from Elsevier.

1. Now, get down on the ground and kneel on one knee. Place the ball under the shin of the kneeling leg, as far down the leg toward the ankle as you can without letting the ball roll out from under you.

2. Proceed slowly over the ball and up the shin until the ball stops moving at the bone below the knee joint. Mark on your PFA any painful areas in this shin muscle (anterior tibialis).

3. Lie facedown on the floor, place the ball just above the kneecap, and slowly proceed up the front of the thigh (quadriceps) back toward the hip and pelvis (not toward the groin and pubic bone). You will likely find areas of tenderness and tightness here; many athletes have tight quadriceps from frequent squatting and running activities.

4. Continue slowly rolling in a straight line until you bump into a prominence on your pelvis bone (just above where your thigh joins the trunk), called the anterior superior iliac spine. This is one of two bony points in the front of the pelvis, one on each side of the lower abdomen. Since the hip flexor tendons attach here, this is a common site of tenderness and tightness in athletes who do lots of activities on their legs. Remember to mark any sore areas on your assessment sheet.

5. Repeat on the opposite leg.

Deep Front Line

The deep front line (DFL; figure 4.4, *d* and *e*) defines the myofascial core of the body. It begins deep in the underside of the foot, passes up behind the bones of the lower leg and behind the knee to the inside of the thigh, and in front of the hip joint, pelvis, and the lumbar spine. It continues around and through the thoracic viscera, ending on the underside of the cranium.

Keep in mind that even though this is called the deep front line, it is three dimensional and therefore has volume. Yet, it acts functionally like a continuous line, from foot to head, in the sense that it is all connected. When it gets out of balance there are repercussions, large and small, anywhere and everywhere up and down any of the fascial lines. As such, the DFL harbors much of the chronic sources of inflexibility, decreased athleticism, and pain.

In this assessment, you follow the line from the inside of the calf and thigh to the groin.

1. Lying on your belly, raise your head and upper body, propping yourself up on both forearms.

2. Keeping one leg extended, bring the other hip and knee up about 45 degrees or to where it is comfortable, keeping the lower leg and foot relaxed and loose. (This is kind of like the way soldiers crawl, by raising one leg up about 45 degrees in order to plant and power fulcrum off the knee.) Place the ball on the inside calf of the bent leg as far down toward the ankle as you can without letting the ball slip away. Proceed over the ball slowly, using your upper body strength to push and roll your body backward over the ball.

3. Move the ball up the inner calf until it stops below the knee joint. Then place it above the knee joint and continue up the center of your inner thigh, but also moving slightly off the center line in different directions,

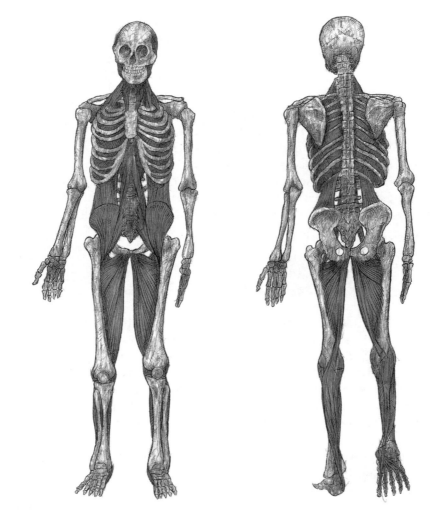

Figure 4.4d-e   The deep front line (DFL).

Reprinted from *Anatomy trains*, T. Myers, p. 190, 2001, with permission from Elsevier.

until the ball ends high up at the tendons of the groin. You may also assess the tissue in varied directions around the groin tendons, obviously avoiding any pressure on the genitals. This is especially beneficial for athletes who have torn or strained their groin in the past and have lots of scar tissue still present. Or they may have injured their knees by spraining the medial collateral ligament (commonly known as the MCL) and have had compensatory tightness in the hip adductors and groin.

4. Repeat on the opposite leg.

5. Skip over the delicate area that includes the entire abdomen and the bottom of your breastbone. Still lying facedown, let one arm rest on the ground in front of you, bent at the elbow, palm down, with the forearm

supporting the weight of your forehead. Let the other arm lie comfortably out to the side, where it will act like an outrigger, helping to direct you over the ball. (Remember that these hand, arm, and head positions are only general guidelines. Experiment with these positions to find out what works best for you.)

6. Place the ball in front of your body in the area of your pectoral muscles—between the shoulder joint and the breastbone. In men the ball should be below the collarbone and above the nipple; in women below the collarbone and above the breast. Just stay within this area and slowly creep and crawl your body over the ball along the floor, searching for tight and tender points and then marking the most significant ones on your PFA sheet. This region is usually much tighter on the side of the dominant arm, especially in throwing athletes who have overtrained these muscles. Remember to not roll directly over any ribs (thick muscles like the pectorals and back muscles usually protect the ribs enough) or areas that make you hurt or stop breathing. You might also want to use a pillow to support your head and neck when working on the upper body.

Now examine all the areas in which you've identified trigger points on your evaluation form. These are some of the prime regions that are likely causing faulty and restrictive movement patterns for you. With this map of your signs and symptoms, you are well on your way to eliminating many of these problems. Doing so will immediately improve not only your strength and flexibility but also, even more importantly, the proper firing activation and sequencing of the muscle fibers that had trigger points. Improving this alone will boost athletic performance.

Step 7: Review Your Findings

Now that you have completed the first six steps of the PFA, what you end up with are several body maps showing your symptoms and assessed movements. When our clients take the time to document, study, and reflect on their personal physical history as it is displayed in the form of personal body maps, the way they feel when they compete and train starts to make more sense. Their maps show so much about their bodies: what has happened in the past, what is happening now, and even what may happen in the future. Such a body map can become a valuable asset in any athlete's ongoing pursuit of excellence.

One of the best ways we've found to use these maps, is to relate them to the fascial lines. You can do this by comparing the personal body maps created in your PFA with the illustrations of the fascial lines shown in figures 4.4, *a* through *e*. We walk you through an example of such a comparison in the next chapter as you learn how to use the findings you gathered to develop an effective individualized flexibility program.

Personal Flexibility Assessment

Name _____ Date _____

History

See pages 50 to 51.

    A. List any injuries, surgeries, or physical problems you have experienced in the past. If more than one, list them chronologically, starting with the most recent.

    B. List any current health problems, complaints, injuries, or current diagnoses made by a health professional.

Symptoms

See page 51. Describe what you are feeling in terms of soreness, tightness, pain, or any other discomfort during daily activities or athletic performance.

Posture and Alignment

See pages 52 to 56. List here all areas that you can see that are out of alignment, (e.g., lower shoulder, higher hip, rotated foot).

From *Stretch to Win* by Ann Frederick and Chris Frederick, 2006, Champaign, IL: Human Kinetics. © Stretch to Win Systems.

Mark on the body map diagrams any areas that are out of alignment. Note any obvious bends, tilts, rotations, and shifts.

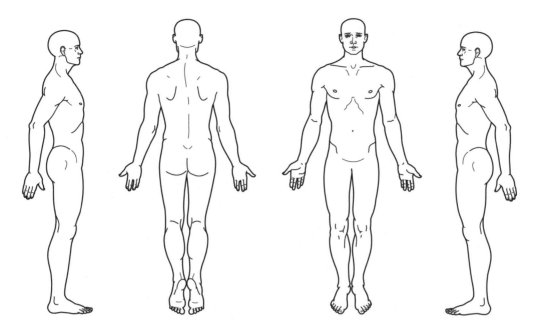

Sport-Specific Movement

See pages 56 to 57. Select several body positions your sport requires. List them here and then describe how you feel getting into and out of these positions.

Choose a dynamic sport movement for your sport and note below how smooth it feels when you perform this movement.

Active Range of Motion (AROM)

See pages 57 to 67 and perform all of these movements in front of a mirror. Note where restrictions are in your active range of motion for each test:

1. General spine
   Flexion
   Extension
   Side bending
   Full body rotation

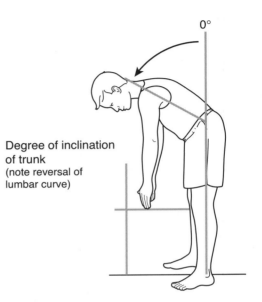

Degree of inclination
of trunk
(note reversal of
lumbar curve)

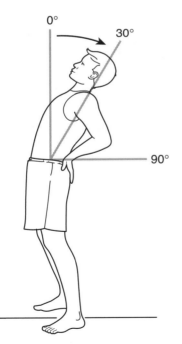

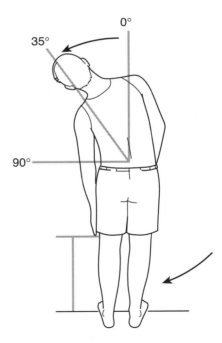

From *Stretch to Win* by Ann Frederick and Chris Frederick, 2006, Champaign, IL: Human Kinetics. © Stretch to Win Systems.

2. Upper extremity
   Flexion and extension
   Abduction and adduction
   External and internal rotation
   Reach behind back

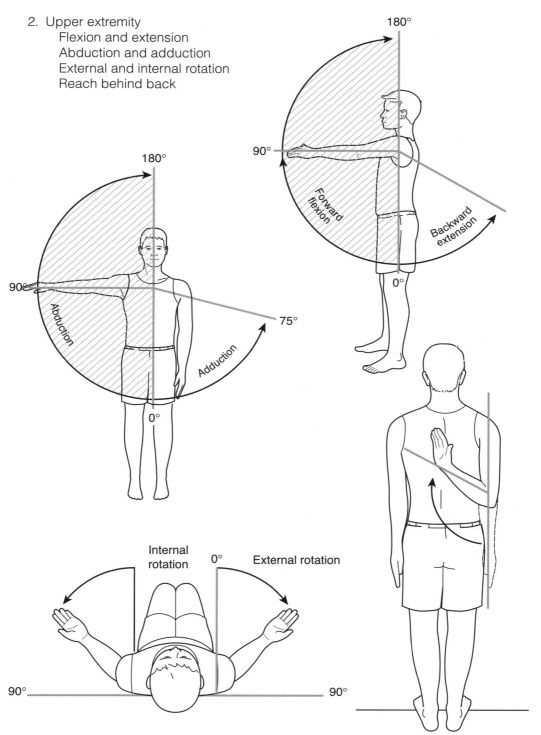

From *Stretch to Win* by Ann Frederick and Chris Frederick, 2006, Champaign, IL: Human Kinetics. © Stretch to Win Systems.

3. Lower extremity
   Standing hip flexion, right and left
   Standing hip extension, right and left
   Standing hip abduction, lateral lunge right and left
   Standing hip adduction, lateral lunge right and left
   Standing hip rotation, right and left

4. Combination movements
   Spine
   Upper extremity
   Lower extremity

Trigger Points

See pages 67 to 75. List below the trigger points you have found. Mark the body diagrams with an X to show where on the body you have located your trigger points.

Review Findings

Review your findings and note them here. Look for correlations between your past and current histories and any present areas of complaint that may be impacting your athletic performance. For example, are the trigger points that you have found located on or near regions that are bothersome or that do not move well?

   Keep this as a record of self-evaluation so that you may repeat it in one week to document your progress.

chapter 5

Your Customized Program

In helping you to develop your own flexibility training program, we begin with several considerations. First and foremost is using the information you've learned from completing your own personal flexibility assessment (PFA) detailed in the previous chapter.

As you learned in chapter 1, in order for a flexibility program to have maximal impact, it should be developed with your individual needs in mind (see principle 10, page 14). To accomplish specific performance goals, you will need to set specific parameters for achieving them. Yet these training parameters must have built-in adaptability so that you can easily modify them if any conditions change. With your completed PFA in hand, it's time to figure out what your PFA has identified as areas to work on. That will help you determine what your individual goals are for your flexibility training program. At that point you can decide what parameters you want to follow, and then develop your own program.

Based on our experience, a flexibility program should do the following to be most effective:

1. It should rapidly and effectively prepare you for and help you recover from any activity.

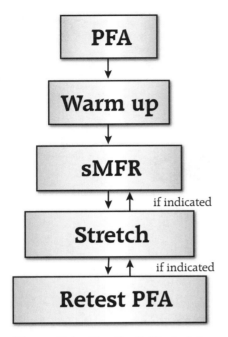

PFA

↓

Warm up

↓

sMFR

↓↑ if indicated

Stretch

↓↑ if indicated

Retest PFA

Figure 5.1 The flexibility training progression.

2. It should integrate and not conflict with your current program of strengthening and conditioning as well as all other aspects of training and competition. This means it is adaptable enough to always fit in with your current training schedule.

3. It should specifically prepare you for the intended activity and serve your individual flexibility needs.

4. It should provide you with an accurate and individualized system that helps you periodically reevaluate how you feel and move so that you can manage your own progress.

Figure 5.1 shows the general progression of developing your flexibility training program, from the PFA to the warm-up preparation for sMFR to the stretches and back to the PFA again to retest what felt tight or was restricted in motion.

Interpreting Your PFA

Your completed PFA immediately gives you answers about what is currently affecting your flexibility (and other aspects of your performance) and gives you direction for addressing your flexibility imbalances on your own before they become big problems. After you follow the guidelines of your PFA and begin self-treatment, you will get results. These results in turn will help you decide how much self-treatment and maintenance you need to achieve balanced, optimal movement—called homeokinesis—for your sport or activity. Anytime you lack homeokinesis, reassess your flexibility needs through a PFA to find out why you are out of balance. By managing your training in this manner, identifying and eliminating small problems before they become big ones, you will make faster and better progress in reaching your athletic goals without complications. Consequently, your flexibility program will take only as much time as you need to reachieve balanced, optimal movement appropriate to your sport or activity.

Performing a PFA and adjusting your program accordingly brings big payoffs in how you feel and perform in your sport. And the program doesn't have to add much time to your current schedule. In fact, it will actually save you time because you won't need to visit the athletic trainer or schedule appointments to see other professionals for most of the problems that arise; you will often be able to identify and treat yourself (though, as we've said, you do need to see a doctor or other practitioner when you are unable to quickly resolve the problem yourself).

Your PFA should now consist of a thorough personal history of your subjective complaints, problems, injuries, and surgeries; an evaluation of your posture, created as you analyzed yourself in a mirror; a body map marked with trigger points and other areas of tightness that you discovered when rolling on the balls; and an assessment of simple movement patterns in the form of active range of motion (AROM) of major joints and muscles.

One of the best ways to use your findings to optimize your flexibility training is to compare the body maps from your completed PFA to the fascial lines in figure 4.4, *a* through *e*, to see how you can design an optimal follow-up flexibility training program based on your individual needs.

To walk you through an assessment review, we'll use the sample PFAs shown on pages 84 to 88. In this example for Susan S. you see the following:

History. Swimmer's shoulder (rotator cuff tendinitis)

Symptoms. Pain in right shoulder after swimming.

Posture. Head shifted forward; lifted right shoulder; increased lordotic curve in the low back.

Sport movement test. Susan complains of slight tightness and pinching in the right shoulder when simulating the overhead movement that her arm makes when swimming "the crawl."

Active ROM. Decreased right external and internal rotation; decreased abduction and flexion.

Trigger points (TP). Right shoulder blade; right upper back; right shoulder top and front.

Now let's see how Susan's symptoms correlate with particular fascial lines.

- Her body map clearly shows where her TPs are; later in this chapter you'll learn how she can use sMFR to eliminate them. Since she has four TPs—two on the front of the right shoulder girdle and two on the back—we know that they directly affect at least these parts of the superficial front line (SFL) and superficial back line (SBL). But, as we learned in chapter 2 about tensegrity, if one part of the line is affected, the whole line is involved. Therefore, for optimal results, Susan should spend some time exploring the whole fascial line (and other intersecting lines) to eliminate these TPs; doing so will allow her to connect the dots and see how one part of her body in one location can cause pain or dysfunction in another, seemingly unrelated location. In truth, all of the fascial lines (and there are others that are not discussed in this book) are more or less affected by anything that is structurally misaligned or maladjusted in the body because each line is part of one integrated fascial system.

Personal Flexibility Assessment— Sample A

Name _Susan S._   Date _12/15/06_

History

See pages 50 to 51.

A. List any injuries, surgeries, or physical problems you have experienced in the past. If more than one, list them chronologically, starting with the most recent.

none

B. List any current health problems, complaints, injuries, or current diagnoses made by a health professional.

swimmer's shoulder
(rotator cuff tendinitis)

Symptoms

See page 51. Describe what you are feeling in terms of soreness, tightness, pain, or any other discomfort during daily activities or athletic performance.

pain in right shoulder after swimming

Posture and Alignment

See pages 52 to 56. List here all areas that you can see that are out of alignment, (e.g., lower shoulder, higher hip, rotated foot).

head shifted forward
higher right shoulder
increased curve in low back

Mark on the body map diagrams any areas that are out of alignment. Note any obvious bends, tilts, rotations, and shifts.

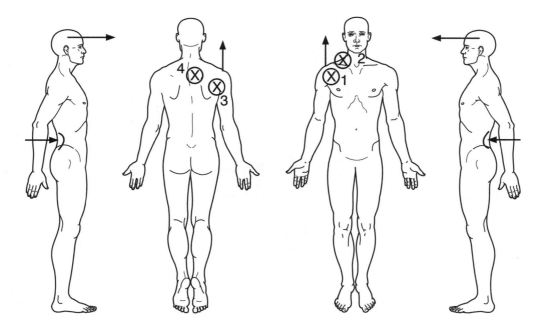

Sport-Specific Movement

See pages 56 to 57. Select several body positions your sport requires. List them here and then describe how you feel getting into and out of these positions.

> *slight tightness in right shoulder with*
> *overhead swimming motion*

Choose a dynamic sport movement for your sport and note below how smooth it feels when you perform this movement.

> *pulling through swim position pinches in*
> *shoulder*

Active Range of Motion (AROM)

See pages 57 to 67 and perform all of these movements in front of a mirror. Note where restrictions are in your active range of motion for each test:

1. General spine
   Flexion
   Extension   } *normal range*
   Side bending   *of motion*
   Full body rotation

0°

Degree of inclination
of trunk
(note reversal of
lumbar curve)

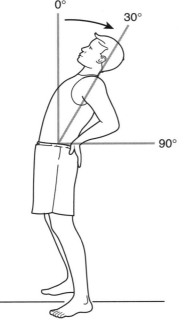

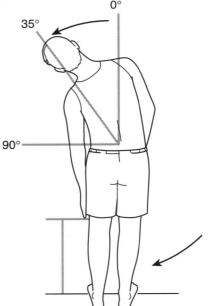

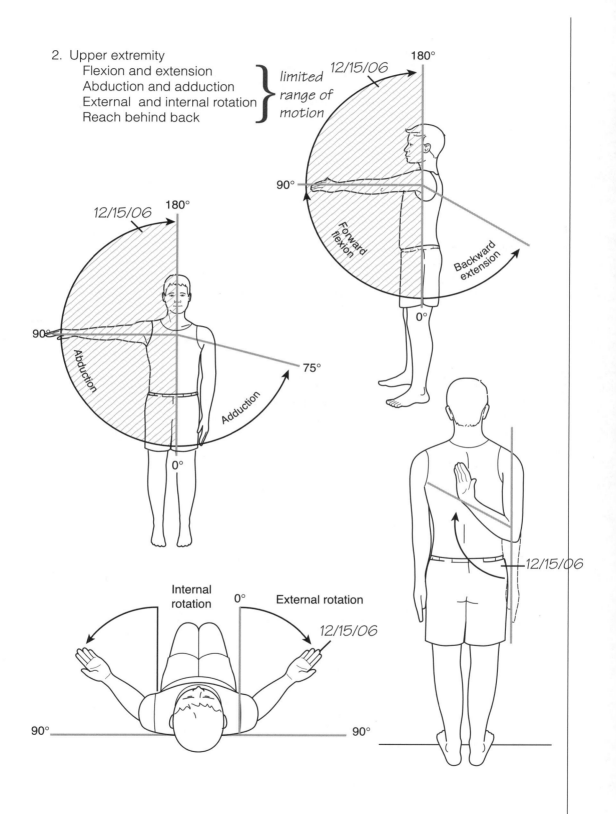

2. Upper extremity
   Flexion and extension
   Abduction and adduction   } limited
   External and internal rotation   } range of
   Reach behind back   } motion

12/15/06

180°

90°

0°

Forward flexion

Backward extension

12/15/06

180°

90°

75°

Abduction

Adduction

0°

Internal rotation

0°

External rotation

12/15/06

90°

90°

12/15/06

3. Lower extremity
   Standing hip flexion, right and left
   Standing hip extension, right and left
   Standing hip abduction, lateral lunge right and left
   Standing hip adduction, lateral lunge right and left
   Standing hip rotation, right and left

   all normal

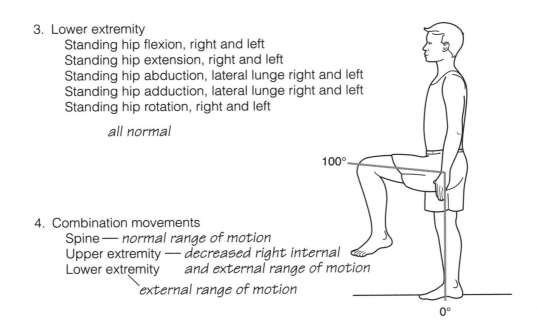

4. Combination movements
   Spine — *normal range of motion*
   Upper extremity — *decreased right internal*
   Lower extremity   *and external range of motion*
                external range of motion

Trigger Points

See pages 67 to 75. List below the trigger points you have found. Mark the body diagrams with an X to show where on the body you have located your trigger points.

1. *front of shoulder*   3. *shoulder blade*

2. *top of shoulder*   4. *upper back—right side*

Review Findings

Review your findings and note them here. Look for correlations between your past and current histories and any present areas of complaint that may be impacting your athletic performance. For example, are the trigger points that you have found located on or near regions that are bothersome or that do not move well?

Trigger points are locatd where tightness
and pinching in shoulder occur.

Keep this as a record of self-evaluation so that you may repeat it in one week to document your progress.

- After releasing her trigger points with sMFR, Susan will want to stretch the areas around the TPs and the fascial lines that extend to and from them so that she eliminates not only the TPs, but also the tightness and restricted mobility that comes with them. Guidelines about how to stretch tight regions and the areas that have trigger points can be found in the stretch matrix we describe later in this chapter and in chapter 6.

- Susan will retest the swimming motion and the active range of motion of her restricted shoulder right after her sMFR and stretching to see if her approach was successful. If she was successful, then she will continue to do her PFA once per week to ensure that she is maintaining good recovery from activity. If she is only partially successful, then she may go back to repeat her sMFR and stretching and retest again. She may have rolled over her TPs too fast or not done her stretches long enough; these are two common beginner mistakes. Guidelines for these parameters follow later in this chapter.

On pages 90 through 94 we see the example of Kevin K., whose PFA points to some lower body issues.

History. Right knee anterior cruciate ligament (ACL) repair after college football injury 1995; has worn orthotics since 1996.

Symptoms. Right knee pain after running or leg workout and tight right hip.

Posture. Lower right shoulder; higher right hip; right knee slightly bows in and forward.

Sport movement test. Kevin plays quarterback (QB) in flag football league and is a triathlete. When he does the QB drop and shuffle to his right, he feels discomfort and tightness in his knee joint and outside thigh.

Active ROM. Decreased right hip flexion, extension, and abduction associated with a feeling of tightness as compared to the left.

Trigger points (TPs). Right hip flexor (tensor fascia lata, or TFL) radiating down the iliotibial band; right low back muscle (quadratus lumborum, or QL).

When we correlate Kevin's symptoms and physical signs with the fascial lines that intersect them we see the following:

- His major TP is located along the superficial front line (SFL) and lateral line (LL) of the right hip and leg. Another, in his back, is associated with the back of the deep front line (DFL). Although he discovered other less intense TPs while rolling on the ball, these were not addressed at this time.

- After releasing his trigger points with sMFR, Kevin will want to stretch the areas around the TPs and the fascial lines that extend to and from

Personal Flexibility Assessment– Sample B

Name _Kevin K._   Date _1/15/07_

History

See pages 50 to 51.

A. List any injuries, surgeries, or physical problems you have experienced in the past. If more than one, list them chronologically, starting with the most recent.

> *1996—started wearing orthotics*
>
> *1995—right knee anterior cruciate ligament repair*

B. List any current health problems, complaints, injuries, or current diagnoses made by a health professional.

> *2006—right knee strain*

Symptoms

See page 51. Describe what you are feeling in terms of soreness, tightness, pain, or any other discomfort during daily activities or athletic performance.

> *knee pain after running or leg workout*
>
> *tight right hip*

Posture and Alignment

See pages 52 to 56. List here all areas that you can see that are out of alignment, (e.g., lower shoulder, higher hip, rotated foot).

> *lower right shoulder*
>
> *higher right hip/waist*
>
> *right knee tilts inward*

Mark on the body map diagrams any areas that are out of alignment. Note any obvious bends, tilts, rotations, and shifts.

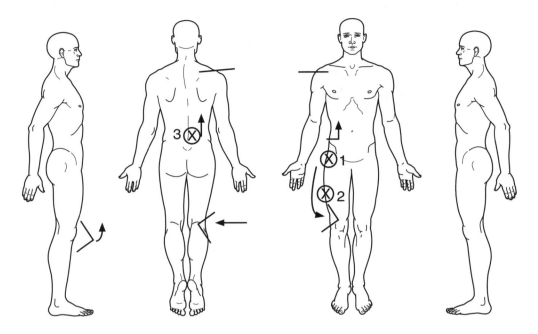

Sport-Specific Movement

See pages 56 to 57. Select several body positions your sport requires. List them here and then describe how you feel getting into and out of these positions.

Right knee tight and stiff in warm-ups, sore after flag football & lower body weight training

Choose a dynamic sport movement for your sport and note below how smooth it feels when you perform this movement.

I play quarterback in flag football. After the snap, my shuffle back to the right is not smooth—I don't always trust the right knee & am afraid I'll twist it too much.

Active Range of Motion (AROM)

See pages 57 to 67 and perform all of these movements in front of a mirror. Note where restrictions are in your active range of motion for each test:

1. General spine
   Flexion
   Extension
   Side bending
   Full body rotation
   } *normal range of motion*

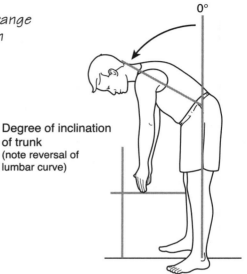

Degree of inclination
of trunk
(note reversal of
lumbar curve)

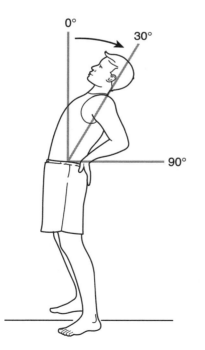

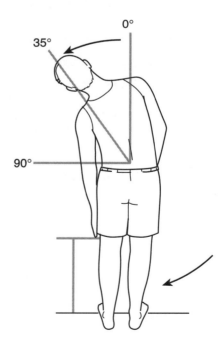

2. Upper extremity
   Flexion and extension
   Abduction and adduction   } *normal range*
   External and internal rotation } *of motion*
   Reach behind back

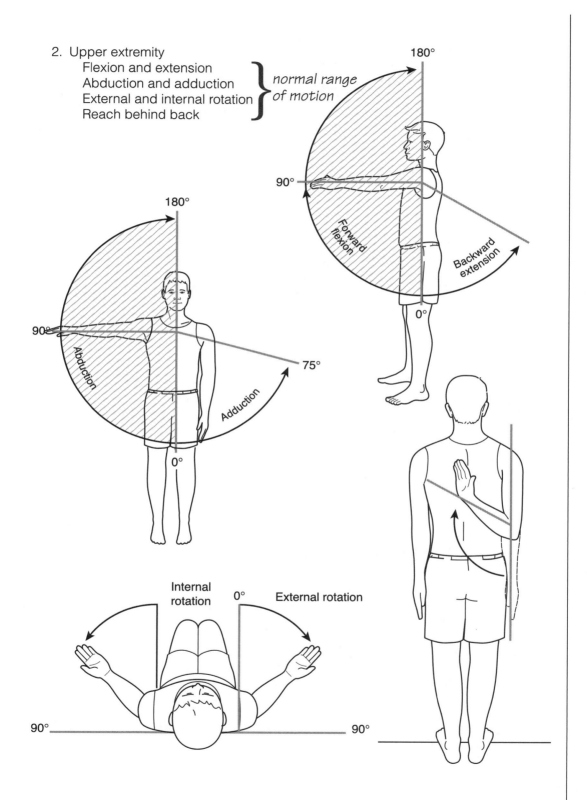

180°

90°

Forward flexion

Backward extension

0°

180°

90°

Abduction

Adduction

75°

0°

Internal rotation

0°

External rotation

90°

90°

3. Lower extremity
   Standing hip flexion, (right) and left   *decreased*
   Standing hip extension, (right) and left   *decreased*
   Standing hip abduction, lateral lunge right and (left) *decreased*
   Standing hip adduction, lateral lunge right and left
   Standing hip rotation, right and left

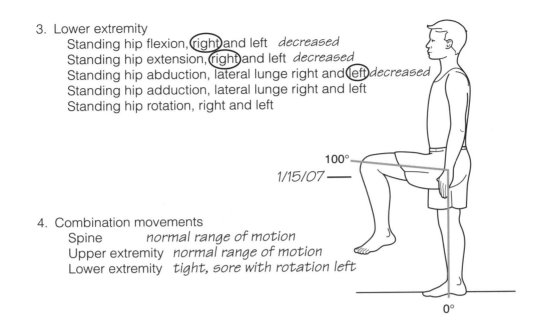

100°

1/15/07 ——

0°

4. Combination movements
   Spine   *normal range of motion*
   Upper extremity *normal range of motion*
   Lower extremity *tight, sore with rotation left*

Trigger Points

See pages 67 to 75. List below the trigger points you have found. Mark the body diagrams with an X to show where on the body you have located your trigger points.

1. *Right hip flexor*
2. *IT band*
3. *Right low back*

Review Findings

Review your findings and note them here. Look for correlations between your past and current histories and any present areas of complaint that may be impacting your athletic performance. For example, are the trigger points that you have found located on or near regions that are bothersome or that do not move well?

> *Trigger point from right hip flexor and IT band*
> *duplicates knee tightness/soreness I feel*
> *when training and playing football.*

Keep this as a record of self-evaluation so that you may repeat it in one week to document your progress.

them so that he eliminates not only the TPs, but also the tightness and restricted mobility that comes with them. Guidelines about how to stretch tight regions and the areas that have trigger points can be found in the stretch matrix we describe later in this chapter and in chapter 6.

- Kevin will retest his sport movements—dropping back and shuffling right for football and testing his running—to determine if his program of sMFR and stretching has eliminated all or most of his barriers to optimal performance. If problems persist, he'll see the appropriate professional for a diagnostic work-up.

These two examples show you how to develop the framework of a flexibility training program from the information you collected your PFA, based on your own physical findings and subjective statements. Take some time now to interpret your own PFA findings to set your own flexibility goals

To go from this framework phase to the concrete phase of a stretching program you need to know more about specific training parameters (such as intensity, frequency, and duration) and whether the flexibility goals are for preactivity or postactivity. We discuss how to consider those factors in relation to your own goals and needs later in this chapter.

Warming Up
With Self-Myofascial Release

In chapter 4 (pages 67 to 75) you learned how to roll on a ball (or foam roll) to locate and identify trigger points and other local sources of tightness in your muscle and fascia. In this section we show you how to eliminate or greatly reduce the presence of these problem areas in your body.

It is always a good idea to warm up the body before doing any type of self-myofascial release or stretching. This holds true even when the stretching itself is considered part of a warm-up. Performing two to five minutes of aerobic activity such as jogging or stationary cycling is enough to get the blood circulating and to warm the tissues.

The process of releasing soft tissue restrictions in the body begins deep in the matrix of the connective tissue. So, after performing aerobic exercise to raise the body's core temperature, for the very best results we recommend also warming up for stretching by using a technique called self-myofascial release (sMFR).

An athlete performs sMFR by lying on a 5- to 7-inch (12- to 18-cm) diameter ball on the floor (or standing with one foot on a tennis ball or on a Footsie Roller if working the feet). The position of the ball depends on which part of the body you are trying to release. Cheryl Soleway, a physiotherapist from Canada and a marvelous teacher, introduced us to this powerful approach. The pressure of the ball stretches as it stimulates, creating space between connective tissue, muscle attachments, blood vessels, and fascia. All the athletes we work with who are truly intent on achieving the most flexibility possible practice this part of their training on a daily basis.

Rolling on the ball can help you reduce or eliminate conditions that can impair your strength and flexibility such as trigger points, scar tissue, and tight spots in the muscles. Active range of motion, strength, and stretching all improve after eliminating these trouble spots in the muscle, as you will see when you retest the restrictions that you identified in your PFA.

When you perform sMFR before stretching, you dramatically increase your flexibility and range of motion. Tension and trigger points in the fascia can hinder the success of a stretching program and limit freedom of movement, which can adversely affect performance. With self-myofascial release the tissue warms up from the pressure and from your movement over the ball, becoming more pliable and able to change its shape. As it lengthens tissues, sMFR also relaxes the tension in the coils of the wavy collagen fibers within them, similar to the effect of a deep massage. This all contributes to greater gains in flexibility and mobility. Of course, there is no substitute for good bodywork from an experienced therapist when you need it. However, sMFR does allow you to work on your own tissues, and it puts you in complete control of the work.

Self-Myofascial Release—Anytime!

There are many ways that sMFR can be incorporated into your program, not just as part of your warm-up. It makes any stretching that follows it more productive and relaxing. You can benefit by taking a minute or so to use it on any specific problem area before a practice or training session. It can even be used to quickly release a couple of spots that might feel tight in the middle of working out. You can perform it as a stand-alone session during the day for any amount of time, from a few minutes to over an hour. The end of the day is an excellent time for sMFR, because it allows you to restore length and balance to your muscles and fascia. It also prepares your body for some deeper stretching before you go to bed. It is a great way to calm down your nervous system and puts you in a perfect state to get a restful night's sleep. When you wake up the next morning, you'll feel more balanced, loose, and ready for action.

The application of sMFR is an extremely helpful adjunct to stretching. Although it is not a mandatory practice, we strongly recommend making it a regular part of your flexibility training program because of its cumulative long-term benefits. We suggest trying to get in at least a couple of areas every day and a full-body sMFR once a week. If you are pressed for time, check out the quick three key spots routine (pages 100-101), which just about anyone can fit into a busy schedule once a week.

Choose Your Tools

There are a number of tools you can use for sMFR, including FitBALL Body Therapy Balls, various foam rollers, Footsie Rollers, The Stick, Thera Canes, tennis balls, and golf balls (figure 5.2, *a* and *b*). You might want to try all of these tools to find out which ones work best for you.

Foam rolls are popularly used for working on tight areas and trigger points but we find that 5-, 6-, and 7-inch (13-, 15-, and 18-cm) FitBalls works well for most people, both because of the three-dimensional qualities of the ball and because users can control the firmness by filling them up with more air or letting some out. How much change you will experience in the fascia using these balls depends on the amount of pressure applied, how long it is applied, and how quickly or gradually it is applied.

The largest (7-in or 13-cm diameter) ball works best for beginners and for people who are 6 feet, 6 inches tall or taller (198 cm) or who weigh 200 pounds (90.8 kg) or more. People whose muscles are extremely tight or tender to the touch or who have many trigger points in their bodies would do well to start with this size. This ball works best for a gentle and general response and release.

The 6-inch (15 cm) ball is recommended for intermediate and experienced participants in sMFR who are comfortable with the work and not currently suffering from any major pain or soreness in their tissue. These balls works best for broad areas of the body, such as the quads and lats, and for people who are heavier in body type.

The smallest (5-in or 13-cm) ball is more intense and is recommended for more advanced and isolated work. It can be used in smaller regions—deep in the hip flexors or rotator cuff, for example. Because of their dense muscular structures

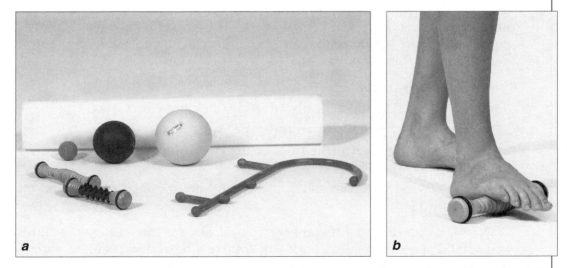

a   *b*

Figure 5.2 Tools for self-myofascial release (*a*) include the foam roll, a self-myofascial release ball, a racquet ball, a tennis ball, Footsie Rollers, and a Theracane. The Footsie Roller (*b*) is an effective tool for breaking up adhesions and releasing trigger points in the sole of the foot.

and enthusiastic attitudes, many of the athletes we work with jump right into using the 5-inch balls, but actually it is better for any athlete to slowly work his or her way toward using them after working on the larger balls. If moving too quickly or exerting pressure too deeply during sMFR causes pain or unnecessary discomfort, there may be a guarding and tightening response in the body. This inhibits the releasing process and is counterproductive. The best approach is to go slowly and be patient as you relax and breathe, working with the ball rather than against it. In the beginning, take many breaks off the ball until you get used to doing it regularly. You can move to a smaller ball as your tissue sensitivity to the pressure decreases. As with your stretching, this is a journey of discovery and not a race to the end!

Remember that the sensation you feel from performing sMFR should never be one of pain, but more a feeling of pressure, then a slight burning or stinging and eventual relief as your tissues relax. This feeling of local fascial stretching and tissue elongating over the ball is very different from the sensations you get from stretching without using the ball. If you detect any significant discomfort that does not subside within a few breaths, it's best to move off the sensitive area and instead work around it, slowly working toward it and retesting pressure on it. Many times this indirect approach lessens the sensitivity enough to allow the area to be worked on. If you experience pain that is intense or that does not subside after the third attempt, immediately move off that spot. You may have gone over a bruised area, a nerve caught in the connective tissue, an area of inflammation, or a bone. Consult a health care practitioner if you have any concerns.

If you ever feel dizzy, light headed, or nauseated, please stop your sMFR immediately. Also, note that a few areas of the body are vulnerable to injury if excessive pressure is applied to them, so be very careful and gentle as you work near or around these regions:

- The coccyx (tailbone)
- The lower 11th and 12th ribs (floating ribs) in the back area
- The xyphoid process (lower tip of the breastbone)
- The abdominal area (the front of the body from the pubic bone up to just below the ribs)
- The cervical vertebrae and upper cervical area (cranial-vertebral nerves, arteries)

Do not engage in sMFR if you have any stitches, fractures, or open wounds. You should also not engage in it if you are receiving anticoagulant therapy or might be suffering from any of the following disorders: malignancy; osteoporosis; osteomyelitis; acute rheumatoid arthritis; inflammatory conditions; systemic or localized infection; sensitive diabetes; hypersensitive skin conditions; or circulatory conditions (e.g., edema, hematoma, or blood pressure problems).

Self-Myofascial Release Routines

You'll want to return to pages 69 and 74 to review the myofascial lines that the routines follow. In *Anatomy Trains*, Tom Myers writes "Muscles operate across functionally integrated body-wide continuities within the fascial webbing. These sheets and lines follow the warp and weft of the body's connective tissue fabric, forming traceable 'meridians' of myofascia. Strain, tension, fixation, compensations, and most movement are all distributed along these lines."

When you look at the body from this integrated perspective, you can see more clearly how crucial it is to achieve and maintain as much freedom of movement as possible. It is especially important because, as Myers points out, the interconnectedness of the myofascial lines, or meridians, makes a lack of flexibility anywhere in the body a problem for the entire body. Athletes need bodywide freedom of movement in order to perform at their highest potential.

Sample Self-Myofascial Release Schedule

Refer to your PFA to see which areas of your body are tight and tender, then plan your weekly sMFR program accordingly. A typical program would include the following:

Feet	Two or three minutes	Daily
Three key spots	Five to ten minutes	3 x per week
Full program	Up to one hour	1 x per week

As you perform self-myofascial release, keep the following tips in mind:

- Breathe. Exhale into the tissue and relax as you move through the area.
- Think about moving in three dimensions, that is, thoroughly explore each area that you are rolling on.
- If you come upon a tender spot, reduce the pressure you are applying and try to stay in that place for several deep breaths until the tenderness lessens. If the tenderness does not decrease, keep moving.
- If you find a tight spot, stay at that point for a few seconds until you feel the tissue releasing.
- The speed at which you choose to move helps determine the intensity of the work. The general rule is that the more slowly you move, the more intense the sensation will be, but, often, the greater the tissue release will be as well.

FEET

As the literal foundation of the body, the feet are involved in most athletic movement. They have one of the highest concentrations of nerve endings in the entire body, and working on them can be a quick and powerful way to release tension throughout the body. For foot rolling you can use a tennis, racquet or golf ball, but we prefer something called a Footsie Roller, which is a 6.5-inch (17-cm) round wooden object that we have been using for over 30 years.

1. Stand facing a wall or stable object that you can use for support. Place the Footsie Roller or ball in the center of your heel and begin to put some of your weight on it.
2. Slowly roll it toward the toes, pulling the roller or ball toward you as you roll. Apply as much pressure as you can tolerate. Stop when you feel any tightness or tenderness and wait until it releases or lessens before continuing.
3. Once you get to the tips of the toes, reverse directions and roll slowly back down to the heel.
4. Place the roller on the outer edge of the foot and repeat steps 1 through 3, moving from the heel to the toes and back down again.
5. Place the roller on the inside edge of the foot and repeat steps 1 through 3, moving from the heel to the toes and back down again.
6. If you feel that the tissues of your foot are sufficiently released, perform the full sequence on the other foot.

THREE KEY SPOTS

If you have only 5 to 10 minutes for sMFR, you can choose to target three key spots that are common areas of tension and tightness. Begin with the feet (as described previously), move to the hip and low back area, and then work on the spine. The hip (including the six deep rotators) and low back area is one of the tightest regions in most athletes and is crucial to all athletic movement. Releasing the spine is fundamental to getting the back, shoulders, and neck to open up.

1. Perform the foot self-myofascial release (described in previous exercise).
2. When you are finished with your feet, sit on the floor and place the ball directly in the center between your two sit bones on your sacrum above and off your tailbone. Place your feet flat on the floor and your hands on either side of your body.
3. Slowly move over the ball in this area in small circles, then over to one side of the glutes, staying close to the sit bone, which many muscles attach to. Move back and forth, up and down, and in all directions, targeting the glute tissues and fibers. The deeper you sink in this area the more of the six deep rotators you will reach.
4. To target the lateral side of the hip and back, slowly turn onto the hip with the ball beneath your side, placing your forearm on the floor to support yourself. Roll around in this area, again moving in all directions, on the lateral fibers of the hip.

5. Move the ball up toward the rib cage (being careful not to put pressure on the floating ribs) and make contact with the tissue of the quadratus lumborum, which is in your waist area.

6. Continue turning over until you are facing the floor, with the ball under your hip flexor area, and roll around in all directions.

7. Return to the original sitting position with the ball underneath you, and repeat steps 3 through 6 on the other hip.

8. When you've finished the hip series on both sides, it's time to move on to your low back. Lie on your back with the ball beneath your sacrum and your legs slightly bent, feet on the floor.

9. Roll back and forth with the ball on sacrum, moving out to the sacroiliac joint on both sides. Be careful not to put pressure on your tailbone (coccyx).

10. Move in all directions on the low back. To increase pressure, lift both feet off the floor if you can and continue moving in small circles, supporting and stabilizing yourself on both forearms.

11. With the ball still under the sacrum, put the feet on the floor hip-width apart, keeping your legs slightly bent. Interlace your fingers and place hands behind your head.

12. Use the legs to assist your movement by walking and pushing and pulling off the feet as you roll over the ball.

13. Slowly roll up over the ball along the center of your spine. Extend or arch the trunk by relaxing it as you roll over the ball from the bottom of the spine to the top of the neck.

14. Release the hands and spread the arms out to each side on the floor as you increase the trunk extension and feel the chest opening up to prepare for the next move.

15. Interlace the fingers and place them behind the head again and roll the ball down the center of the spine, using trunk flexion to increase the feeling.

16. Move the ball just off to one side of your spine and roll it back up to the neck. Roll it back down again on the same side of the spine.

17. Repeat on the other side, upward and downward.

FULL PROGRAM

If you have more time, you can expand the program to target the whole body. Start with the three key spots routine and continue down the other lines as follows.

1. After you finish the three key spots program, you'll move down to the back of your lower body. To begin, lie on your back and place the ball below the sacrum. Place the palms on the floor beside the hips and use the hands to control the pressure of weight bearing, taking care again not to put pressure on the coccyx. Roll the ball down the glutes, hamstrings, and calf on one side and back up again. Repeat on the other side.

2. Lie on your side with the ball underneath you to get at the lower body lateral line. Roll from the bottom of the rib cage (avoiding pressure on the actual rib) for the QL, across the gluteus medius, down over the center of the lateral aspect of the thigh for the ITB and peroneals. Moving slightly to the front will get the lateral quads and moving slightly to the back will get the lateral hamstrings as both of these muscles attach to the IT band. Roll back along the same line in the opposite direction, if desired. Repeat on the other side.

3. Turn your body over so that the chest and hips face the floor. Bend one knee and place the ball up inside the groin on one side to target the lower body inside line. Roll the ball down the inside of your thigh, moving over the adductors and down to the medial gastrocnemius. Repeat on the other side. The inner thigh is usually a tender area and it is usually quite sensitive, so proceed slowly and with caution.

4. Target the lower body front line by placing the ball in the front of the hip joint area, keeping to one side and below the abdomen, and rolling down through the quads. You can increase the intensity by bending the knee and grabbing the foot with the hand on the same side as the bent leg, if you are able.

5. Now it's time to continue with the lateral line through the torso to the upper body. Lie on your side, extending your arm straight up, so that it is in line with your body. Place the ball beneath the origin of the latissimus dorsi on the lateral-posterior crest of the hip. Slowly roll up toward the shoulder and the teres major and onto the rotator cuff tendon, on the side of your shoulder blade. After you finish this area, place the ball on the side of the neck down by the base and roll it up to the base of the head, avoiding rolling anywhere near the front of the neck. Repeat on the other side.

6. You'll finish by working with the upper body front line. Turn your body so that the chest and hips face the floor and place the ball on one side of your chest to do the pectoralis major (working around but not on the breast in women), and then out toward the shoulder along pectoralis minor. Next, rotate your head toward the opposite shoulder and roll up the side of your neck up to the base of your skull. If you cannot rotate your head in this position, eliminate the neck and finish with the shoulder. Repeat on the other side of the body.

Understanding Stretching Parameters

Before you decide what types of stretching best suit your needs, it's important to understand the parameters that make a stretch effective. You must be aware of the intensity, duration, and frequency of a stretch before you can incorporate it into a safe and effective flexibility program that complements your current training.

How strongly you feel a stretch is a subjective evaluation of **intensity** that can range from not feeling much of anything (a very mild stretch) to feeling a lot of pain (a maximal stretch). In our program, the intensity of any given stretch is regulated by your breathing, and we recommend that every stretch be pain free. You know you're stretching with too much intensity if you stop breathing during a stretch or feel like you want to stop breathing, if you feel pain or a very strong sensation of pulling in the muscles being stretched, or if you feel that your muscles are getting tighter or starting to "lock up." Signs that you are stretching with just the right amount of intensity include the following: finding yourself breathing deeply, fully, and with satisfaction (you may even yawn); experiencing a feeling of release in the regions being stretched; and moving farther into the movement or stretch without effort.

Usually, the **duration** of a stretch refers to the time (in seconds) for which you hold the stretch; in chapter 1 we discuss the drawbacks of timing a stretch in seconds. Later in this chapter you will learn how the way you breathe affects the rhythm and tempo of a stretch. If you keep the quality of your breathing high, you'll naturally hold the stretch for the proper duration.

The **frequency** of a stretch refers to the number of times you repeat it, within one stretch session or within another time frame such as a day or week. The proper frequency for any particular stretch depends on how much release has occurred in the myofascia after you've followed the guidelines for intensity and duration. You can test this actively and functionally after performing a stretch by trying to assume the positions or perform the movements that give you trouble in the form of soreness, lack of mobility, or suboptimal flow of movement. Your range of motion in these positions may have improved greatly, moderately, or not at all. If you find only slight improvement, simply repeat the sequence of stretches until you achieve greater range of motion (or as time permits). If you start feeling like you're getting tighter, you may not have been paying enough attention to the signals in your body and as a result may have exceeded the proper intensity or duration of the stretch. Or you may have something else going on such as being dehydrated.

We have found that if you become more aware of your response when you breathe appropriately during a stretch, the parameters of intensity, duration, and frequency are immediately and spontaneously set at an optimal level. Your stretching will be much more efficient if you are aware of your breathing and the subsequent response of your body than if you focus on attempting to meet predetermined parameters. We have found that the effect of stretching with

Reasons Not to Stretch

- Lack of joint stability (e.g., because of a recent sprain or fracture)
- Endangered vascular integrity due to diseases or drugs (e.g., anticoagulants) that weaken or otherwise alter vascular structure or function
- Infection or inflammation in or around involved structures
- Acute injury—scar tissue must have formed before you can stretch safely
- Diseases that affect the condition of the tissue targeted to be stretched
- Excessive pain or other negative reactions to stretching
- Lack of compliance with a program because of not tolerating or desiring the procedure

Modified from Mühlemann and Cimino 1990.

awareness is cumulative so that after approximately four weeks of this kind of stretching, you will find that you have made more progress more quickly and with less effort than you would with a traditional stretching program.

Range of motion (ROM) is conventionally thought of as the total motion available to a joint as determined by the way the bones that make up that joint move in a specific direction. It may be an estimated measurement or it may be a more precise one determined by using a tool called a goniometer. Both active range of motion (AROM) and passive range of motion (PROM) can be measured. AROM is determined when an athlete moves his or her body, limb, or head to the limit of a defined movement; PROM is determined when someone else moves the athlete's relaxed limb or body through the limit of a defined movement. Common limits to movement include muscle tightness, joint stiffness, muscle spasm, joint inflammation, and pain. The ROM of some heavily muscled athletes is limited by the bulk of the muscle. For instance, the increased girth in their shoulder girdles and arms may make them unable to reach and scratch their backs. PROM is almost always greater than AROM, because the latter is limited by contracting tissue that curtails movement. Generally, contractile tissue does not limit PROM except when there is tightness, increased muscle bulk, or other problems.

Stretching is the act of increasing ROM by elongating tissues that have a tendency to get shortened or compressed (we discuss the causes and effects of these tendencies in chapter 2). Our target tissue is the myofascia, which may be stretched both actively and passively, as explained later in this chapter.

Traditional Stretching

While there are other designations and divisions, stretching has most commonly been divided into three general types: static, dynamic, and ballistic. Static stretching is best for increasing static or passive flexibility, or PROM; dynamic stretching is best for increasing dynamic or active flexibility, or AROM; and ballistic stretching (defined farther on in this section) is best for increasing ballistic flexibility, a specific kind of flexibility used in such sudden, quick, high-powered movements as swinging, throwing, or jumping.

While these terms can mean different things to people in different professions, for most, static stretching involves holding a position, whether the athlete holds it him- or herself or someone else assists. We have discovered that this concept of "holding" a stretch prevents many athletes from making progress with their flexibility. When we ask first-time clients to demonstrate to us their concept of a static stretch, they often hold the position so rigidly and with so much effort and control that there is no possibility for the relaxation response to occur. Athletes also tend to hold their breath when they stretch this way, thereby increasing tension in the body. While one of the intentions behind static stretching is to relax the muscles, it can have the opposite effect, as we've seen with many clients who have not had much success in increasing their flexibility through assisted or self-static stretching. The failure of holding a position to produce gains in flexibility is also reflected in the scientific and medical literature. For these reasons, and also because one meaning of "static" is "motionless; not moving or changing," we prefer not to use the term "static stretching." We prefer a different term that allows for movement within stillness during a stretch, which we discuss in the next section.

Dynamic stretching (sometimes incorrectly used interchangeably with ballistic stretching) is performed without holding positions. A dynamic stretch takes a joint through its active range of motion while the person stretching performs controlled, often "swinging" movements. Good training programs often include dynamic stretching within their general warm-ups, but it may also be used in individualized warm-ups that target specific areas of the body that are going to be worked, such as the shoulders and torso of a pole vaulter or the torso and hips of a gymnast who is about to do the pommel horse routine.

Ballistic stretching, on the other hand, according to the National Strength and Conditioning Association (NSCA 2002) "typically involves active muscular effort and uses a bouncing-type movement in which the end position is not held." Ballistic stretching may also include a more intense or higher-amplitude form of dynamic stretching like leg swinging, or it may include plyometric exercises such as bounding or depth jumps, which are designed to enable a muscle to reach maximal force in the shortest possible time.

Undulating Stretching

Rather than use the three traditional stretching terms—static, dynamic, and ballistic—we like to use the term *undulating* to describe more clearly the types of stretching we recommend. All our stretches fall along a continuum of undulating stretching, from very slow to very fast undulations that, like traditional stretching, may be done actively or passively with assistance.

The word *undulating* means rising and falling like a wave, a metaphor that, we think, illustrates an effective way to stretch. Anyone who has been to a seaside beach has seen how an ocean wave rolls up onto the beach and then retreats back toward the ocean at a predictable tempo. Sometimes this tempo is slow, calm, and barely detectable—as on a windless afternoon, for example. Other times, such as during a windy storm, it is fast and furious. An example of an athletic counterpart to the movement of an ocean wave is a jump that has an initial "fall" or squat in the preparatory prejump phase, then a "rise" during which the athlete accelerates to the peak distance or height, then another "fall" with the descent and landing phase.

As a feature of program design and planning, the characteristic or quality of undulation is also used in strength training as in "undulating periodization," a nonlinear-based training system, which many trainers claim is superior to traditional linear systems in terms of strength gains (see Rhea et al. 2002). Anything that undulates has an inherent quality of flexibility; this is a characteristic of dynamic living systems. That is why things like your respiratory rate, heart rate, and blood pressure are not constant. They are always in flux, because that is how living systems respond to the stimuli inside and outside the body.

There are many examples of undulating or wavelike motions in the body. Breathing is the first that comes to mind. When you break down the physical act of breathing into its components, you see that it involves a coordinated series of movements in the rib cage, abdomen, spine, sacrum, pelvis, legs, shoulders, arms, cranial bones, and internal organs. The sequence of movements in all these areas that occurs when you breathe is the natural wave or undulation of the body. Stretching can be viewed similarly. We like to call undulating stretching "doing the stretch wave"—the image of an undulating wave not only corresponds to an effective way to stretch but also suggests how to synchronize your breathing with the stretching movements (see chapter 1, page 2, principle 1, "Synchronize your breathing with your movement"). Synchronizing your breathing with the stretch movement, as opposed to "holding" a static stretch, will allow you to release into the stretch and thus help you optimally elongate the tissues you are stretching.

By performing undulating stretching, you avoid the recontracting and retightening of the area just stretched that is quite common in traditional stretching. This is because the wave itself is accomplished by using different firing patterns that move the muscles into and out of the stretch positions. If a stretch feels too strong, release it for a moment and gently wave back into it again. If you are not feeling a stretch in the targeted area, it could be because you are so tight in other areas that you cannot get the selected area to stretch, or maybe your body position is incorrect. If you can't feel a stretch but your body alignment is correct and nothing elsewhere in your body is restricting you, then you actually may have sufficient flexibility in that area. It does happen occasionally!

Two basic traits of undulating stretching form the basis of our entire Stretch to Win system: the alternating flow quality of the movement and the tempo of the movement, which can span the spectrum from very slow to very fast.

Alternating Flow

The alternating flow of a movement is a rise-and-fall, a back-and-forth, or an oscillation that occurs throughout the stretch and is initiated and maintained by regulating one's breathing. You can experience this by trying the following stretch. This exercise works especially well when you perform it cold (i.e., when you are not warmed up).

1. Stand with the feet about shoulder-width apart and comfortably parallel.
2. Inhale deeply as you lift the top of the head (not the chin) toward the ceiling.
3. Exhale as you drop the chin down toward the chest.
4. Continue breathing normally as you let the head and arms drop forward, releasing the shoulders, the upper back, and then the lower back. Go as far down as your body comfortably lets you, keeping the knees relatively straight but not locked.
5. When you reach the bottom of the movement, inhale and exhale. Then start very slowly rolling back up vertebra by vertebra.
6. Repeat five times very slowly.

With each repetition, feel how the body rises a little with the inhalation and falls a little with the exhalation, both while you are in motion and when you pause in the fully bent-over position. This is the natural undulation or wave motion of the body as you breathe, the motion within stillness when you perform the stretch wave very slowly. If you forcefully try to reach your hands to your toes or to the ground as in traditional static stretching, you constrict your breathing and stop the undulation from occurring. This defeats the purpose of the stretch, which is to increase your mobility. If you let your breathing initiate and complete the movement, you will notice by the fifth repetition how much you can increase your flexibility without forcing it.

To feel another example, try the following:

1. Lie flat on your back with the legs straight out in front of you and the arms down by your sides.
2. Bend the right knee up toward the chest, bringing the foot off the floor, and interlace the fingers behind the thigh. Let the leg relax down into your clasped fingers, with the elbows toward the floor.
3. Keeping the hands clasped behind the thigh and below the knee, inhale as you extend the knee away from the chest until the elbows straighten; let the knee straighten as far as is comfortable. (If you do not feel comfortable in this position then you are very tight and should stop this exercise now, skipping over the next two steps to the paragraph that follows them.)
4. Gently pull the entire leg up to the chest, until you feel the first bit of resistance to the movement.

5. Stop at that point where you feel the stretch and bend the knee again. Repeat the same sequence five times.

Notice how, once you are coordinating this movement, the rise and fall of the leg movement harmonizes with your breathing for a painless progressive stretch through a full range of motion.

Tempo

The tempo is the timing or rhythm of the stretching movement. We divide stretch waves into four different tempos: very slow, slow, fast, and very fast. Since breathing is what initiates the wave of movement in your body as you stretch using our system, we use one complete breath cycle—one inhalation and one exhalation—as the measure of tempo in stretching the wave.

Stretch wave very slow (SW_{VS}) = three very slow breaths per stretch position

Stretch wave slow (SW_S) = two slow breaths per stretch position

Stretch wave fast (SW_F) = one regular breath per stretch position

Stretch wave very fast (SW_{VF}) = one fast breath per stretch position

We use these categories to help simplify and categorize the tempos, but in reality you'll find the right tempo for each stretch you do based on your own experience and what you are trying to accomplish with it. Just as in resistance training, in stretching we choose different tempos for different reasons and goals.

Choosing Your Tempo

Using the breathing process in stretching is certainly not a new concept, but we think we employ a unique method of using the breathing to direct the stretch. In our system, for example, instead of counting for the typical 10 seconds, you take three slow and relaxed breaths while allowing the body to undulate in the stretch position. If at the end of those three deep breaths your body isn't letting go and releasing the targeted area, then you take two or more additional breaths until you feel the tension relax.

In other words, as an alternative to letting almighty time dictate how long you hold a stretch, you can listen to your body and use your breath to inform you of what feels tight. If you follow your breath and the feeling of the tissues being released, you might do a stretch for 5 seconds. For another person the stretch may take 10 seconds, and for yet another person it might take 20 seconds. The point is that you want to hear what your body is telling you in the present moment. We have found (clinically, with assisted stretching and in the field, with active stretching) listening to the body to be a more accurate guide than the arbitrary times that many conventional stretching programs dictate.

Therefore, when a client asks, "How long should I do this stretch for?" our response is always "For as many breaths as it takes to get the tissues to let go."

Notice that we say tissues, not muscles, because there are so many layers of different connective tissues involved.

The most effective way to use your breath in stretching is to move into the stretch on your exhalation and gently release the stretch on your inhalation, allowing the breath to move through the body like a wave. Move as smoothly as possible through each stretch, visualizing your body as a wave and moving it like one. The movements within each stretch might include rotating and bending side to side as well as moving up and down and into and out of the stretch wave. Remember to let the breath direct and guide you as to how long you remain in each stretch. The number of breaths you take will depend on how and what you are feeling in your body at the moment that you decide to stretch. On some days both sides of your body may feel quite equal, and on other days you might notice a significant difference in tightness between one side and the other. If this happens, you'll need to spend a bit more time breathing into and stretching the area that feels more restricted. The time you spend stretching depends on your specific needs and goals. The general rule is to take as many breaths as needed until you feel the tissue release before moving on to the next area.

Recall principle 2 from chapter 1, "Tune your nervous system to current conditions." Our aim is to create an ideal state of athletic awareness, which begins with synchronized breathing to condition your nervous system for what you want to accomplish. The body responds powerfully to different tempos of breathing.

Stretch Wave—Very Slow (SW$_{VS}$)

Very slow tempo stretching helps you achieve your most dramatic and permanent gains in flexibility. It is similar to what has traditionally been called static stretching in that when you perform it you do the stretch wave in one position for a prolonged period of time (generally three very slow breaths). The difference is that instead of trying to hold the stretch, you focus on releasing all the tension in your body, undulating the stretch with each slow breath to get maximal tissue elongation in broad or specific areas. By breathing and stretching very slowly—the tempo is slow, the duration is long, and the intensity is initially low—you stimulate your parasympathetic nervous system (see chapter 2). This is what we mean by "movement within the stillness" of a stretch. With muscle tone and tension at a minimum, conditions are perfect for achieving plastic changes (permanent lengthening) in the fascia.

Because the purpose of this particular stretch wave is to take your flexibility to another level by changing the plasticity of the connective tissue in your body, it is best for athletes to perform it during the off-season when they are more relaxed and tend to have more time. During the off-season, professional and high-level athletes are better able to tolerate and recover from the increases in duration and intensity that lead to gains in plasticity. They can achieve and adjust to the improvements in strength, speed, and agility that result from this type of work in the off-season. Then they can reap the benefits of their off-season work while using their in-season stretching to maintain the elasticity of their connective tissues.

When you do the SW_{VS}, take your time with each breath to feel and encourage the wave of movement extend throughout the spine, upper body, lower body, and limbs, no matter what you are stretching. To get the most out of this type of stretching, do a full body sMFR on one day early in the week, followed by a stretching program for the entire body at least twice during the week. Do targeted sMFR and stretches to body regions (upper versus lower body) on those days that you have trained or exercised following your workout. So, for example, if during the off-season you are lifting weights three times per week and running twice per week, you can do full body sMFR once per week and stretching twice per week on off-training days and do much briefer, targeted stretches on the days that you have trained either the upper or lower body.

If you are just coming off an in-season in which you worked particular parts of your body very hard, then we recommend that you use the off-season to make flexibility gains a priority throughout the entire body but especially in those areas that may be prone to increased scar tissue and trigger points. For instance, if you were a punter or kicker in American football, within the time that you have set aside for doing the full body sMFR and stretching routine twice per week, you will want to give more focus and attention to the back, hip, and leg needed for kicking. After eliminating the cumulative problems of the sport season, you will more easily make the kinds of flexibility gains that you are looking for in the off-season. Continue this program until you achieve the desired flexibility as determined by your coaches, your trainers, and your performance on the field. After achieving the required flexibility, switch to a maintenance program of doing the slow stretch wave (SW_S) tempo.

Stretch Wave—Slow (SW_S)

This type of stretching has a slightly faster tempo than the very slow stretch wave, but the breathing is still slow (two slow breaths per stretch), because you continue to want your parasympathetic nervous system to be dominant while you stretch for elastic gains, not plastic gains as in SW_{VS} above. The reason the tempo is faster than SW_{VS} is that the purpose of this type of stretching is to rapidly regain flexibility that has been recently lost. For instance, after a particularly intense day of training, you will either stretch immediately after the activity, while your body core temperature is still elevated, or in the next best case, stretch before retiring for the night, preferably after a warm bath or whirlpool. In our experience, this routine will rapidly get your baseline flexibility back to where it was before you tightened up from training. That means anywhere from 5 to 20 minutes, depending on how tight you are and how familiar you are with doing this routine. Because you are not taking time to do the whole body stretching as in $SW_{VS,}$ you will focus on the body regions that have gotten tight from the day's activities.

For general tightness, stretch all body areas once using this tempo. If you don't feel that you've regained your flexibility after going through the routine, simply go through it again until you have attained the desired flexibility. Athletes know immediately when they've achieved this just by getting up and walking around. Others will usually know after doing a few testing moves like swinging the arms or legs or trying out a sport-specific movement that was previously giving them trouble. For specific areas of tightness, perform all the stretches for that area (see chapter 6) and repeat the sequence during that same stretch session until you reach the desired flexibility.

If you perform SW_S each practice day with the above noted guidelines, you should be fully recovered by the next day. If you find that at the end of the week or toward the middle or end of the season you are having a particularly difficult time staying flexible, then it is essential that you devote some time every week (about one to two hours) to do a full body SW_S program repeating each stretch until the tissue releases the tension or soreness stored within it.

Keep in mind that a slow stretch wave program is appropriate for stretching after workouts, practices, or competition. You can also dedicate entire training sessions to using SW_S to restore flexibility; it can become harder to maintain the flexibility you've attained as the intensity of the athletic season progresses. At these tempos you can perform three or four stretches in five minutes. So if you have 15 minutes, you can select 10 to 12 stretches; 30 minutes gives you time for 20 to 24 stretches; and 60 minutes gives you time for a full restorative session for the whole body.

Stretch Wave–Fast (SW$_F$)

This tempo of stretching helps prepare you for imminent athletic activity (within an hour or two at the most), whether you are training or competing. It is similar to what has traditionally been called dynamic or functional stretching—it too moves the tissues through progressively increasing ROM and uses simultaneous circular movements to warm up the joint capsule—and some form of it may already be part of your current preactivity warm-up. This kind of stretching incorporates waves of movement in multiple planes and directions, rather than just duplicating the paths that your athletic movements will take. This helps prepare your body by stimulating more efficient blood flow to all areas, usually with an additional special focus on the areas that are most important for your specific sport or activity. It also better prepares your joints for movement in all directions by stimulating joint lubrication and joint proprioceptors—those parts of your nervous system on auto-pilot that are responsible for accurately guiding your joints as they move.

In SW_F you breathe at a faster tempo (one fast breath per stretch position) because you want to move at speeds that build up to athletic activity. When you breathe and stretch at this faster tempo you stimulate the sympathetic nervous system. This helps you get optimal recruitment of all the muscles needed for your sport or activity. Doing a 5 to 10 minute sMFR on targeted trigger points then doing the stretch wave fast for 5 to 15 minutes (depending on your needs) before athletic activity will help you to properly warm up your body for sport or athletic activity.

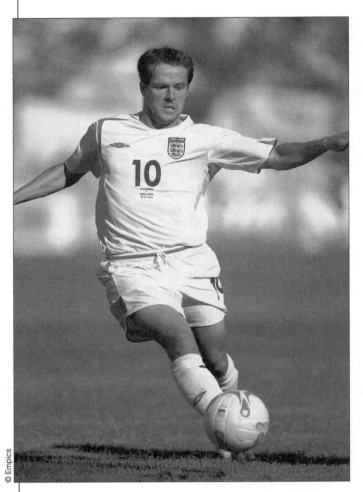

© Empics

Athletes in sports that involve sudden, fast kicking or jumping movements should include some very fast stretch wave work in their training to prepare their bodies for performing such movements in competition.

Stretch Wave— Very Fast (SW$_{VF}$)

This type of stretching incorporates swinging, bounding, jumping, and other fast, aggressive, and intense movements to prepare the athlete for performing these actions in his or her sport. Hurdlers, pole-vaulters, long jumpers, gymnasts, and other athletes who use explosive movements will benefit from an additional warm-up of very fast tempo breathing and movement through the extreme ranges of motion used for their sports.

We recommend performing stretches at the slower tempos first (SW$_{VS}$ in the off-season; SW$_S$ in-season) in order to prepare your body for stretching at the faster tempos. Doing the stretch wave from very slow to very fast at the right time in your athletic season places you on a continuum, gaining passive flexibility before you gain active flexibility. Progressing along this continuum improves your capacity for moving very fast by ensuring that you address all the fundamental aspects of your flexibility that might otherwise cause problems as the season begins and while the season progresses. Too many athletes try to advance their flexibility without first mastering the fundamentals and the result is often injury.

Fast and very fast stretch wave programs are appropriate for use when you have just warmed up (unless such a program is part of your warm-up session), immediately before workouts, practices, and competitions. How many stretches you do can depends on the amount of time you have. For example, you can generally do about 2 or 3 fast stretches per minute, so five minutes would allow you about 10 stretches, 10 minutes would allow you 20 stretches, and 20 minutes would allow you 30 or more stretches (or more repetitions).

Proprioceptive Neuromuscular Facilitation (PNF) Stretching

In chapter 1, principle "Facilitate body reflexes," we describe proprioceptive neuro-muscular facilitation (PNF). Research demonstrates that PNF may offer some of the greatest gains in range of motion.

We use PNF in both our assisted and self-stretching programs. By using stabilizing belts to secure and stabilize one limb during assisted stretching while the other limb has the freedom of undulating stretch movements, the athlete is able to feel get pain relief, eliminate scar tissue and trigger points, and achieve maximal flexibility with ease. During self-stretching, we sometimes have our clients do self-PNF especially when using props like large (55-cm or larger) fitness balls, poles, bands, walls and other objects. This is because they can easily use the prop to hold on to and assist with contracting in the opposite direction of the stretch. Using PNF in particular stretching exercises, is discussed at more length in chapter 6.

In summary, remember that the tempo of your breathing and the stretch wave you choose determine the effect on your nervous system. You might do the same exact stretch routine before an event using a fast stretch wave tempo that you do at the end of the day using a slow tempo to restore flexibility lost during activity. If you pick up the pace you'll be ready for action; if you slow down your tempo you'll be in a more relaxed and calm state.

Selecting Your Stretches

We use the term *matrix* to describe the organizational plan for an athlete's custom-ized stretching program. A matrix provides support or structure to something else, especially in the sense of surrounding or shaping it. Given the fascial matrix that we discuss in chapter 2 and its interconnected role in the body, the term *matrix* seems appropriate for describing how you develop and organize your personal stretching program. While the idea of matrixes based on movement has been around for some time, ours is a bit different in that it can be quite simple or it can be used to put together a more complex stretching program. Like a spider-web, it grows in detail as it expands—as you choose more stretches to add to it. You can decide how basic or how detailed you want it to be. You may choose to focus your stretching on just one small, specific area of the body; on a group of muscles; on a larger region of the body; or on an entire fascial line that connects the lower body and upper body, using a longer series of stretches. You can also choose the matrix that fits your needs based on the amount of time you have available or feel is necessary to spend; it can range from a 5-minute program to a comprehensive 60-minute program. For developing your functional flexibility, the duration of the program is often less important than the flow of the program (figure 5.3, *a* and *b*).

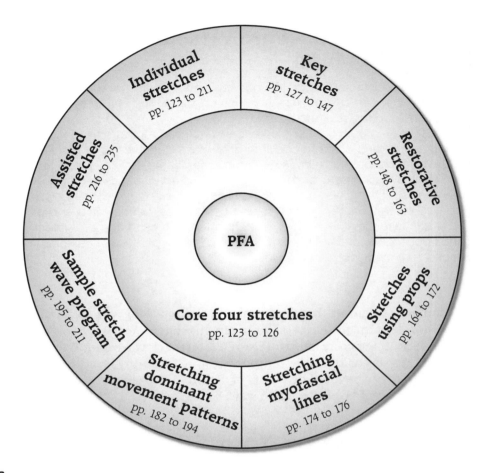

a

Figure 5.3 The Stretch to Win program is centered on assessing your flexibility using the PFA and constructing your routine based on the results. Start with the core four, then pick and choose the stretches detailed in chapters 6 through 8 that suit your needs.

The reason there needs to be such a wide variety of choices in developing a stretching program is that different athletes (and sometimes the same athlete at different times in his or her life) can have many different requirements. A simple program will fit the bill for an athlete who has no serious flexibility problems but just a couple of tight areas that need attention. For an athlete whose lack of flexibility has led to a number of injuries and plagued his or her career, however, a more extensive program is in order. Of course, the more time and attention you dedicate to a flexibility program, the greater the benefit and improvement. If you use only the basic core stretches, it's a good bet that you won't fully realize your body's flexibility potential.

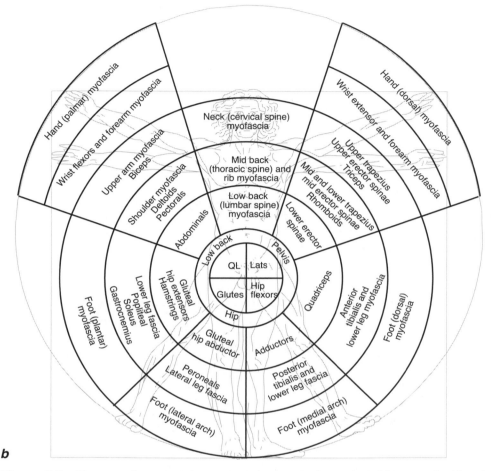

Figure 5.3 The core four stretches are at the heart of our stretching matrix. Use the matrix to determine target areas for your program.

In the next chapter we describe essential stretches for each area of the body, which you can choose from to build your own matrix. From there you can continue to custom-design your program with some of the sport-specific stretches provided in chapter 7 and assisted stretches provided in chapter 8. One of the main goals of this book is to offer more detailed sport-specific stretches and programs than athletes have ever had at their disposal in the past. The more specific the information and techniques you put into your matrix, the more specific the program you can create. With so many options for your changing needs, boredom with your flexibility program will never be an issue. Table 5.1 lists each stretch we describe, the type of program in which it is found, and the area(s) of the body it targets.

Table 5.1 Matrix Stretch Finder

Area(s) of body targeted	Hip flexors	Gluteus complex	Quadratus lumborum (QL)	Latissimus dorsi	Low back-pelvis-hip	Low back and lower erector spinae	Abdominals	Quadriceps	Hip adductors	Gluteal hip abductors
Core four stretches										
Hip flexors, p 124	X				X					
Gluteus complex, p 125		X			X	X				
Quadratus lumborum, p 126			X		X	X				
Latissimus dorsi, p 126				X	X	X				
Key stretches and assisted stretches (second and third page number, when applicable,										
Low back, p 128, 217, 230					X	X				
Gluteus maximus and deep rotators, p 129, 218, 231		X			X					
Gluteus medius, p 129, 219, 232		X							X	
Hip flexors, p 130, 221, 234	X									
QL and TFL and IT band p 130, 222			X							
Latissimus dorsi, p 131, 226				X						
Abdominals, p 131							X			
Quadriceps, p 132								X		
Hamstrings, p 133, 219, 233										
Short adductors, p 134									X	
Long adductors, p 134									X	
Knee-popliteal, p 135										
Soleus, p 135, 220										
Gastrocnemius, p 136, 220										
Tibialis anterior, p 137										
Ankle everters, p 137										
Plantar and toe flexors, p 138										
Dorsiflexors and toe extensors, p 138										
Upper and mid back, p 139, 228										
Rhomboids, p 139, 228										
Shoulder rotators, p 140										
Chest pectorals, p 141, 225										

Gluteal hip extensors, hamstrings	Popliteal, soleus and gastrocnemius	Posterior tibialis and lower leg fascia	Anterior tibialis and lower leg fascia	Peroneals and lateral leg fascia	Foot (planar and dorsal flexors fascia)	Foot (medial)	Foot (lateral)	Neck (anterior, lateral, posterior)	Upper trapezius, erector spinae	Mid and lower traps, erector spinae, rhomboids	Shoulder, deltoids, and pectorals	Upper arm, triceps	Upper arm, biceps	Wrist flexors and forearm fascia	Wrist extensors and forearm fascia	Hands
refer to assisted stretches of same name)																
X																
X																
	X															
	X															
	X	X														
			X													
				X		X										
					X											
					X											
												X	X			
													X			
														X		
														X		

Area(s) of body targeted	Hip flexors	Gluteus complex	Quadratus lumborum (QL)	Latissimus dorsi	Low back-pelvis-hip	Low back and lower erector spinae	Abdominals	Quadriceps	Hip adductors	Gluteal hip abductors
Key stretches and assisted stretches *(continued)*										
Upper trapezius, p 142										
Anterior neck, p 142, 224										
Lateral neck, p 143, 224										
Posterior neck, p 144, 224										
Anterior shoulder, p 144, 225										
Medial shoulder, p 144										
Posterior shoulder, p 145										
Biceps, p 145, 227										
Triceps, p 146										
Forearm and wrist extensors, p 146										
Forearm and wrist flexors, p 147										
Hand, p 148										
Restorative stretches										
Hip warm-up, p 149		X	X	X	X	X				X
Hip openers, p 149	X	X						X		X
Front of hip and torso series, p 150	X						X			
Low back series, p 152		X		X	X	X				X
Hamstring series, p 154		X								
Arm series, p 157										
Hip flexor series, p 160	X		X	X			X	X	X	X
Full fascial stretch, p 162	X	X	X	X	X	X	X	X		X
Stretches using props										
Adductor ball stretch, p 165							X			
Lateral line wall stretch, p 166		X	X	X			X			X
Low back chair stretch, p 167		X	X		X	X				
Glute chair stretch, p 168		X			X					X
Hip flexor chair stretch, p 169	X						X	X		
Soleus and gastroc band stretch, p 172										
Hamstring band stretch, p 170		X								

Gluteal hip extensors, hamstrings	Popliteal, soleus and gastrocnemius	Posterior tibialis and lower leg fascia	Anterior tibialis and lower leg fascia	Peroneals and lateral leg fascia	Foot (planar and dorsal flexors fascia)	Foot (medial)	Foot (lateral)	Neck (anterior, lateral, posterior)	Upper trapezius, erector spinae	Mid and lower traps, erector spinae, rhomboids	Shoulder, deltoids, and pectorals	Upper arm, triceps	Upper arm, biceps	Wrist flexors and forearm fascia	Wrist extensors and forearm fascia	Hands
									X							
								X								
								X								
								X								
											X					
											X					
											X					
													X			
												X				
															X	
														X		
																X
X										X						
X	X				X											
										X	X	X	X			
X	X			X				X	X	X	X	X				
			X				X									
X																
X																
	X			X	X	X	X									
X	X				X											

Area(s) of body targeted	Hip flexors	Gluteus complex	Quadratus lumborum (QL)	Latissimus dorsi	Low back-pelvis-hip	Low back and lower erector spinae	Abdominals	Quadriceps	Hip adductors	Gluteal hip abductors
Myofascial line stretches (second page number, when applicable, refers to assisted										
Front line, p 175	X						X	X		
Back line, p 175		X			X	X				
Lateral line, p 176, 235			X	X	X	X	X	X		X
Deep front line, p 176	X						X	X	X	
Dominant movement patterns										
Low back, p 186		X	X	X	X	X				X
Hamstrings and lower body, p 185		X	X	X	X	X				X
Hip release on all fours, p 187		X	X	X	X	X				X
Standing and prone hip flexors, p 189	X		X	X			X	X		
Sitting hip flexors and quadriceps, p 188	X		X	X			X	X		
Lower legs, p 190		X								
Kicking, p 191		X			X	X				
Integrated hip and arm, p 193	X	X	X	X	X	X	X	X		X
Throwing, p 192	X		X	X	X	X	X		X	X
Sample stretch wave program										
Hip circles, p 196	X	X	X		X				X	X
Leg swings, p 198	X	X	X	X	X	X	X	X	X	X
Hip series—kneeling, p 197	X	X	X	X	X	X	X	X	X	X
Glutes—standing p 200		X			X	X				X
Abdominals, p 200	X						X			
Quadratus lumborum (QL) and iliotibial (IT) band, p 201			X	X			X			X
Low back, p 202		X	X	X	X	X				X
Glutes—lying, p 203		X			X	X				X
Hamstrings, p 204		X			X	X			X	X
Lower legs, p 205		X			X	X				X
Lateral line, p 206			X	X	X	X	X			X
Arm swings, p 207				X			X			
Arm series, p 209										

Gluteal hip extensors, hamstrings	Popliteal, soleus and gastrocnemius	Posterior tibialis and lower leg fascia	Anterior tibialis and lower leg fascia	Peroneals and lateral leg fascia	Foot (planar and dorsal flexors fascia)	Foot (medial)	Foot (lateral)	Neck (anterior, lateral, posterior)	Upper trapezius, erector spinae	Mid and lower traps, erector spinae, rhomboids	Shoulder, deltoids, and pectorals	Upper arm, triceps	Upper arm, biceps	Wrist flexors and forearm fascia	Wrist extensors and forearm fascia	Hands
stretch of same name)																
								X			X			X		X
X		X						X		X	X	X		X		X
			X				X	X		X	X	X	X	X		X
					X			X			X		X	X		X
X										X						
X	X			X	X		X									
											X			X		
X	X	X		X	X											
X	X	X	X	X	X	X	X									
								X	X	X	X	X	X			
X	X			X	X			X	X	X	X	X	X	X	X	X
X																
X	X	X	X	X	X	X	X		X	X	X	X	X	X		
X																
X	X															
			X				X									
X									X							
X																
X	X															
X	X				X											
				X		X	X	X	X	X	X				X	X
								X	X	X	X			X	X	X
										X	X		X	X	X	X

chapter 6

Matrix Stretching Techniques

As you've already learned, our system of stretching is unique; it doesn't always follow conventional thinking. Therefore, before we delve into the actual stretching techniques, let's review a few of the key principles of our system, which we first discussed in chapter 1; you'll apply these principles to the stretches.

An individual muscle is only one part of a structural chain that needs to be addressed when you are stretching. Rather than trying to trying to single a muscle out, think beyond that muscle and visualize stretching the fascia and tissues that connect to it as well (principle 5, page 8). We reiterate this principle here because the reason most stretching programs fail is that they do not address all the factors that limit range of motion (ROM). The body works as a unified system with connective tissue intertwining with and linking all its parts. You really must understand this to attain your true flexibility potential.

Apart from the rectus abdominis, very few tissues in the body (bone, muscle, ligament) are actually linear. However, it is quite common for athletes to stretch in only one direction or plane of motion. To achieve the greatest flexibility in your muscles and fascia you need to play with multiple angles and planes of movement, including components of rotation, spirals, and diagonals, when you stretch (principle 6, page 9). Venturing into these new angles and directions will open up a multitude of new possibilities for your sports performance.

It is best to remain in a stretch for just a little while and then move into different angles, exploring all the possibilities of movement, to target the connective tissue around the entire joint (principle 7, page 11). Once you feel the tightness diminish in one position, change the levels and directions of the stretch. When doing a stretch, especially for the hip or shoulder joint, really work the tissue in all the directions around the joint before moving out toward the extremities. Finally, always think about adding space in the joint as you stretch (principle 8, page 12). This objective is aided greatly by using objects such as a band or doorjamb when stretching. We discuss stretching with these props later in this chapter.

Core Stretches

One of the things we've learned through the years of running our practice is the importance of finding the highest-priority aspect of flexibility for each athlete we work with. Because movement in many sports begins with the hip region, opening the hip area is nearly always the first and most important step in designing a stretching program. Another reason this region needs special attention is that it is often the deepest barrier of tightness that restricts flexibility and reduces efficiency of movement. We find that most of our new clients suffer from tight, or hypomobile, hip joint capsules and restrictive tightness in the multitude of muscles and connective tissues surrounding the hips.

We recommend four core stretches to improve flexibility in the hip region, specifically targeting the hip flexor complex; the gluteus complex, including the six deep rotators; the quadratus lumborum; and the latissimus dorsi. These four stretches make up the foundation of the Stretch to Win matrix. Although we view the body as a completely integrated and interconnected form, it's necessary to approach it practically in terms of the known muscular framework. It is from these crucial areas in and around the hips that the program of stretches is built, beginning with the core stretches and then adding other stretches based on athletes' individual and sport-specific needs.

You can use these four core stretches as the basis for routines that change according to your condition. For example, if you are feeling tight from the day's activity and there is another tough day of training or a game ahead, after performing the core stretches you might consider a more comprehensive program for other areas of the body that need extra attention (we refer to this as a restorative flexibility program; see pages 148 through 163). If time is short and you have to get out there and get moving, performing the four core stretches alone will get your hips ready for action.

Perform this sequence of stretches in a flowing manner—whether you are doing them at a very slow tempo or a very fast tempo—to target the four core areas for movement. Use them alone or as the foundation of your stretching matrix. The effect you desire will determine how much time you spend on your routine.

You can either use these core four stretches or choose other stretches for the hip flexors, glutes, quadratus lumborum, and lats from the key stretches to meet your individual needs. What is important is that you begin any stretching session with stretches that target these four core areas, and if you can combine them so they flow together, this makes for even more effective stretching. Once you have stretched these core areas, you are ready to build out your matrix of stretches to include the extremities.

Perform all the stretches with one leg and arm and then repeat the entire series on the other side.

HIP FLEXOR

1. From standing, kneel in a lunge start position with the right leg back. Inhale, keeping the chest lifted and abdominal muscles pulled slightly inward. Exhale and lunge, pressing the right hip forward until you feel a slight stretch. Inhale and release the stretch and your body slightly. Then wave into the stretch on the exhalation again. Repeat the stretch wave as many times as necessary, using the breathing pattern just described, until you feel the tissue release.

2. To progress the stretch along the front fascial line, inhale and reach the right arm upward, then exhale, lunging into the stretch wave and maintaining a lifted torso and slightly arched back. Drop your arm and inhale as you release the stretch and return to start position.

3. To progress the stretch into the lateral line of the hips and torso, inhale then exhale as you lean the upper body over to your left side while at the same time gently pushing your hips out to the right. Inhale as you release the stretch and return to start position.

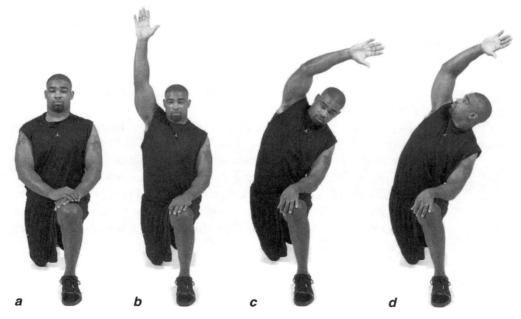

a　　　　　*b*　　　　　*c*　　　　　*d*

4. From the leaning position, rotate the torso by turning the chest upward. Reach the right hand upward and turn the palm to the ceiling. Experiment with the angles of your arm as you exhale.

5. Repeat until you feel all the tissues are moving freely. You may feel this stretch in the front of the hip of the leg pointed back, in one or both groins, in the back, in the opposite hip, and in the shoulder of the raised arm.

GLUTEUS COMPLEX

1. From the lunge position, drop your buttocks to the floor and bring the front foot inward until the foot touches the other knee.

2. Place the hands in front of you in a push-up position with the arms straight. Inhale and lengthen the torso from the top of the head.

3. Exhale as you lower the upper body over the front knee until you feel a slight stretch, then wave back up by inhaling and rolling through the spine.

4. Repeat, going lower on each repetition until you can comfortably lower the torso to the floor. Place the head on the hands, feeling the wave of breathing in this position increase the stretch farther.

5. Push yourself slightly upward and outward of the previous position and do the stretch wave to each side alternately, keeping the hands on the floor. This targets more of the low back area in addition to the glutes.

6. Slowly exhale as you look around toward the back leg and walk the hands in that direction until you feel a slight stretch.

7. Look to the front again to relieve the stretch with an inhalation, then exhale as you look toward the back foot, going a little farther each time you repeat this movement. Progressively make larger movements as your body releases the tightness. In doing so, feel different parts of the body respond and stretch based on the angle that seems to be restricted.

As you do this stretch, visualize moving the wave up the spine to the top of the head, lowering the wave down to the floor, and then rolling it back up.

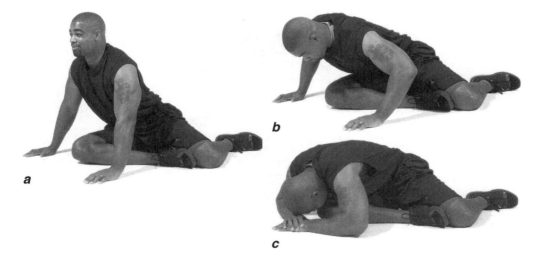

a

b

c

QUADRATUS LUMBORUM

1. Lift the torso up from the last position; again lengthen it outward from the top of the head as you exhale.
2. Drop onto the right forearm and press the left hand into the floor as you exhale to open up the quadratus lumborum and lateral line.

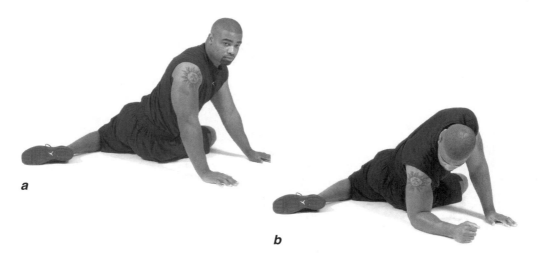

a

b

LATISSIMUS DORSI

1. Inhale from the last position and exhale as you reach the left arm overhead.
2. Rotate the torso, lifting the chest to the ceiling as you exhale, and continue reaching hand outward. Turn the palm upward to face the ceiling.

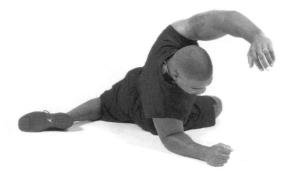

Repeat the entire sequence on the other side by lifting up onto the knees and sliding the other leg forward into a lunge position.

Key Stretches

We have selected the most effective stretches for general flexibility—we refer to them as the key stretches. This is where you start designing your personalized program (after stretching with the core four, of course), using the key stretches as your building blocks. It is best to have a specific order in which to do your stretches—a smooth routine is not only more time efficient, but also necessary for maximizing your flexibility gains (refer to principle 3, page 6).

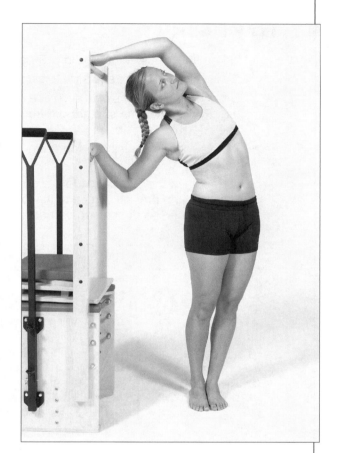

As you'll recall from principle 3, part of following the proper order of stretches is working to open up the single-joint muscle groups before stretching the multiple-joint muscle groups in the hips, legs, shoulders, and arms. One-joint muscles attach right over and near the joint capsule.

After the single-joint muscles and the joint capsule are made more flexible, you can stretch the multi-joint muscles more effectively as the layers of muscle and connective tissue, from deep to superficial, are released in a logical anatomical order.

It is important to stretch from the core, or center, of the body out to the extremities. Stretch the areas that are closest to or within the torso first to loosen the core regions for movement, and then add more stretches to increase flexibility throughout the entire body. Think of the all the stretches as being connected, linked together like the steps to a dance.

As you build your own matrix, add stretches that extend out to the edges of your current range of motion. For example, moving the opposite arm overhead when doing a leg stretch will increase the fascial pull.

LOW BACK

1. Lie on your back, exhale, and pull both knees into the chest.
2. Rock back and forth and side to side while hugging the knees.
3. Drop the knees to one side and slide the top leg slightly forward over the bottom leg. Place the arms straight out from the body on the floor to help keep the shoulders on the floor.
4. Exhale, as you press the top knee down toward the floor with the opposite hand.
5. To increase the stretch, slide the bottom leg as far away from the top leg as possible and press the knee of the top leg to the floor, keeping both shoulders on the floor. The bottom leg can be straightened to increase the stretch.

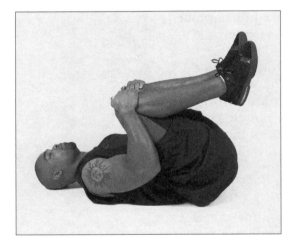

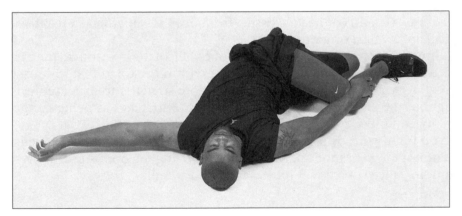

GLUTEUS MAXIMUS AND DEEP ROTATORS

1. Still lying on your back, place both feet flat on the floor with knees bent.
2. Place right ankle on the opposite knee with the hands supporting the knee and ankle.
3. Inhale, then exhale as you push the right knee away from the body to target the hip flexors and deep rotators of the leg. Repeat as needed.
4. Next, keeping the right leg at a 90-degree angle, exhale as you pull the right knee toward the center of the chest with one hand on the knee and one hand on the ankle. Pull until you feel the stretch. To increase the stretch, reach through the bottom leg and pull both legs toward the chest.

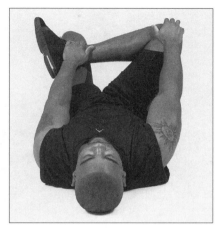

GLUTEUS MEDIUS AND HIP ABDUCTORS

1. From the last position in the previous stretch, bring the knee of the top leg to the center of the body and exhale as you pull it down into the chest.
2. Grab the ankle of the top leg and bring it down toward the floor with the opposite hand.
3. Exhale and roll the body to the opposite side of the crossed leg to increase the stretch.
4. Explore the different angles and fibers by moving around slightly. To increase the stretch, move the knee to the opposite shoulder and pull the ankle to the floor.

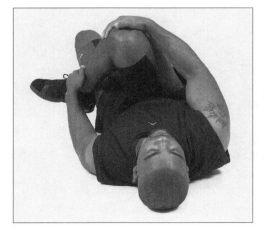
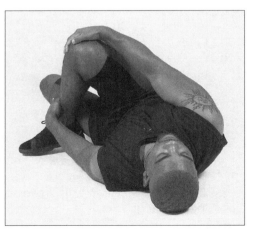

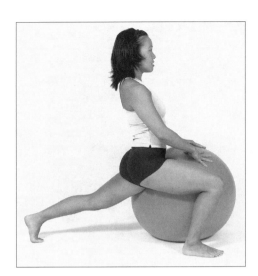

HIP FLEXORS

1. Place a stability ball against a wall. Get into a lunge position with the left hip bone pressing against the ball and the hands on the ball. The ball will help the torso lift upward.

2. Exhale and press into the ball with the hip of the leg that is extended backward, keeping both hips square.

3. Keep the torso lifted upward and pull the abdominals in toward the spine as you gently lean back into extension.

4. Continue to press into the ball with your hip as you slightly move your torso left and right to get different angles of stretch. To increase the stretch, bend back into deeper extension and slide the back leg farther out.

QUADRATUS LUMBORUM AND ILIOTIBIAL BAND

1. Place a stability ball against a wall and lean one side of the torso and hip against the ball. Cross one leg over the other.

2. Slide the bottom leg away from the ball as you lean into ball with the hips and rib cage.

3. Continue leaning into the ball as you lift the torso upward and back toward the bottom leg.

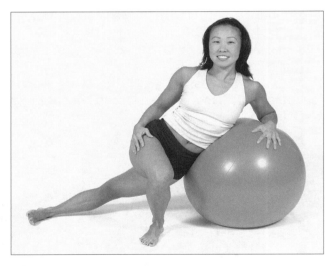

4. Exhale and let the hip on the ball sink downward as you gently rotate the pelvis backward and forward.

5. To increase the stretch, lift the torso upward off the ball and toward the extended leg on the ground.

LATISSIMUS DORSI

1. Find a doorjamb, pole, or other stable object to hold on to. Standing about 2.5 feet (75 cm) from the stable object, inhale and bend laterally at the waist and hips and reach the top arm overhead to grasp the stable object.

2. Exhale and pull the hips away from the object to increase the stretch. To increase the stretch farther, rotate the torso, moving the chest toward the ceiling and then turn the chest toward floor. Explore small changes in movement to feel different regions stretch.

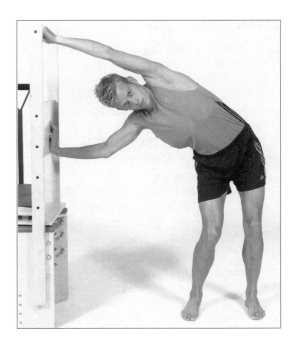

ABDOMINAL MUSCLES

1. Lie facedown on the floor. Inhale, then exhale as you press the hands into the floor, straightening the arms, and lift the upper body upward. Keep pressing the hips into the floor and lengthen the spine through the top of the head.

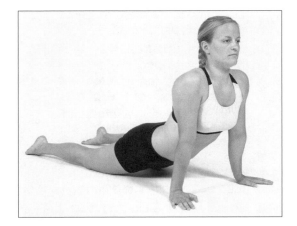

2. As you exhale, lift the upper body as far as possible, but do not allow any pinching in the low back.

3. To increase the stretch, lift the chin to the ceiling. To increase the stretch farther and include the obliques, shift weight more to one hand and look over the opposite shoulder. Repeat the torso rotation to the other side.

QUADRICEPS

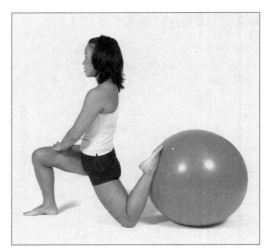

1. Place a stability ball or bench against a wall. From a lunge position, facing away from the wall, place the top of the foot of the back leg on the ball, bench, or other object. Be sure that weight is on the upper knee and not the kneecap.

2. Keep torso lifted up with abdominals pulled in as you arch the back slightly into extension, exhale, and gently push your hips forward.

3. With your back foot still on the ball, roll the ball sideways (or slide the top of the foot) toward the front leg side to target the lateral aspect of the quads. Keep the torso lifted up with abdominals pulled in and the back arched slightly into extension as you continue to gently push the hips forward.

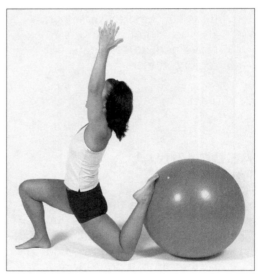

4. Now roll the ball sideways back toward and slightly past the stretched leg to target the medial aspect of the quads. If using a bench, slide the top of the foot on the bench away from the front lunging leg. Again, keep the torso lifted up with the abdominals pulled in and arch the back slightly into extension as you gently push the hips forward.

5. To increase the stretch, reach both arms overhead and arch the back a little more.

HAMSTRINGS

1. Lie on your back with your body relaxed and one knee bent, foot on the floor. Bend the other knee and interlace the fingers behind it, bringing the knee into the chest.

2. Keeping the head and shoulders relaxed on the floor, inhale, then exhale as you gently stretch the leg upward and outward from the joint and then toward the center of chest. Keep the knee bent at this point, focusing on the stretch in the joint.

3. To increase the stretch, with each exhalation, try to bring the leg closer to chest and straighten the knee.

4. Now inhale and gently stretch the leg up and outward from the joint and toward the shoulder on the same side as the stretched leg to work the medial aspect of the hamstring. Again, to increase stretch, try to bring the leg closer to shoulder with each exhalation and straighten the knee.

5. Inhale, then exhale as you take the leg across the body and up toward the opposite shoulder to work the lateral aspect of the muscle. Again, to increase the stretch, try to bring the leg farther across the chest and toward the opposite shoulder chest with each exhalation and straighten the knee.

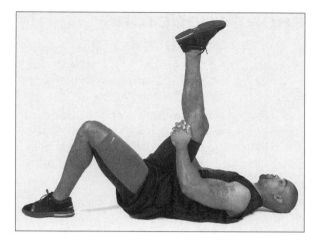

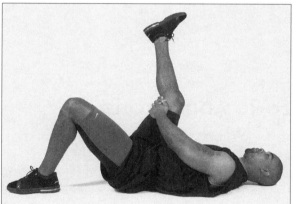

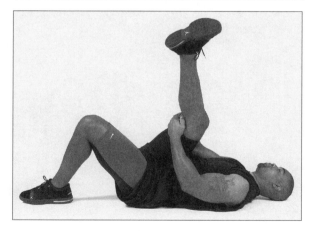

Start with a bent leg and work toward straightening the leg as your flexibility improves over the course of several sessions.

SHORT ADDUCTORS

1. In a lunge position, inhale, then exhale and step the front leg out to a kneeling side lunge until you feel a stretch in the groin or hip flexors (the short adductors).

2. Reduce the intensity of the lunge to decrease the stretch with each inhalation; increase the depth of the lunge or slightly change the foot position to increase the stretch with each exhalation.

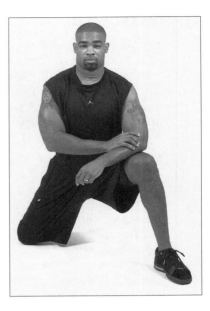

LONG ADDUCTORS

1. To stretch the long adductors from the kneeling position used in the previous stretch, slide one leg out to the side.

2. Try to straighten the knee of the leg being stretched if possible and lean the body forward, relaxing the hips.

3. Change the angle of the stretch by rocking the torso forward and backward; increase the stretch by sliding the legs farther apart so that the body is closer to the floor.

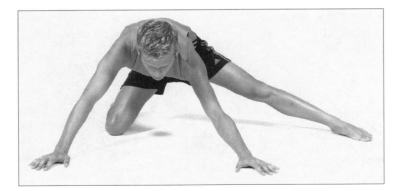

KNEE–POPLITEAL

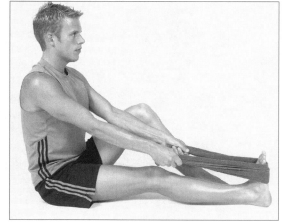

1. You will need a 3-foot (90-centimeter) length of resistance band or a full-size towel. From a sitting position on the floor, extend one leg outward and bend the other leg so that the foot is flat on the floor.

2. Holding one end of the band in each hand, loop the band around the ball of the foot of the straight leg.

3. Sit up tall, exhale, and flex the foot back toward you, using the band to assist the stretch.

4. Slowly slide the heel away from the body as you straighten the knee, gently pressing knee into floor.

5. To increase the stretch, lean forward through the hips with a straight back and flex the foot back closer toward you. This increases the fascial component of the stretch.

SOLEUS

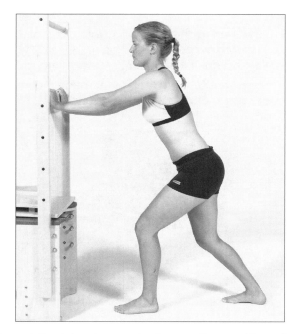

1. Stand 3 feet (90 cm) from a wall or stable surface. Lunge forward, sliding one leg backward and bending the front knee, and rest the hands against the wall or surface.

2. As you exhale, slowly bend the back knee, press the hips toward the stable surface, and keep the back knee bent with the heel on the floor.

3. Slightly straighten both knees to release the stretch and bend them again to stretch.

4. To target the medial aspect of the tissue, change the position of the back foot by rotating the toes outward; to target the lateral aspect, change the position of the back foot by rotating the toes inward. To increase the stretch, increase the bend of the back knee, leaning back into it.

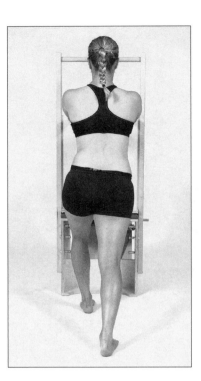

GASTROCNEMIUS

1. Stand 3 feet (90 cm) from a wall or stable surface. Lunge forward, sliding one leg backward and bending the front knee, and rest the hands against the wall or surface.

2. Keep the back foot parallel to the heel of the forward foot and keep the heel of the back foot on the floor.

3. Exhale and press the hips toward the wall as you bend the front knee, keeping the back knee straight.

4. Slightly bend the back knee to release the stretch and straighten it again to stretch.

5. To increase the stretch, contract the gluteal muscles and push the hips more toward the wall.

6. Now rotate the toes of the back foot outward to target the medial aspect of the tissue.

7. Keep the front knee bent and the hips pressing toward the wall. Slightly bend the back knee to release stretch and straighten it again to stretch.

8. Keeping the feet fixed, rotate the hips clockwise, then counterclockwise, to loosen more tissue. Again, to increase stretch, contract your gluteal muscles and push the hips more toward the wall.

9. Now rotate the toes of the back foot inward to target the lateral aspect of the tissue and repeat steps 7 and 8.

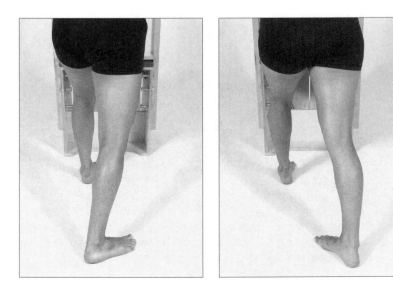

TIBIALIS ANTERIOR

1. From a kneeling position, lean back and place both hands behind you for support. Place the right foot flat on the floor; keep the top of the left foot resting on the floor. (You can use a rolled-up towel or a weight-room pad as a cushion under the top of the foot.)

2. As you exhale, gently rock the left knee up and down. Be careful not to put too much pressure on the top of the foot; direct most of your weight into the hands.

3. To increase the stretch, lift the knee higher off the floor.

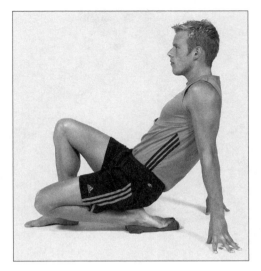

ANKLE EVERTERS

1. Sit in a chair or on the floor; cross one leg over the other above the knee.

2. Gently grab the outside of the foot above the toes, being careful not to twist or compress the toe joints.

3. Stretch the foot up toward the head so that you can see the sole of the foot and feel the stretch in the outer calf, ankle, or foot.

4. To increase the stretch, lift the ankle upward (without lifting the leg) as you continue to move the sole of the foot toward your head.

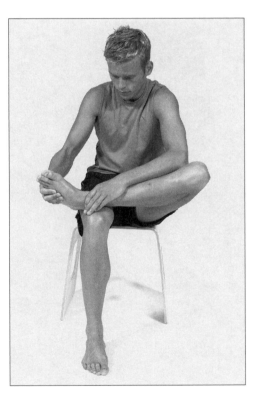

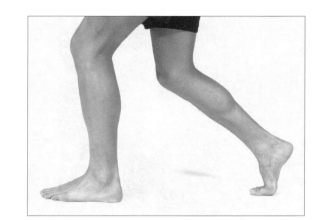

PLANTAR AND TOE FLEXORS

1. From a standing position, slide one foot backward and lift the back heel up off the floor.

2. Bend both knees while pressing the ball of the back foot into the floor.

3. Shift your weight back and forth between the legs to stretch the bottom of the foot.

4. To increase the stretch, bend the knee more as you lift the back heel higher.

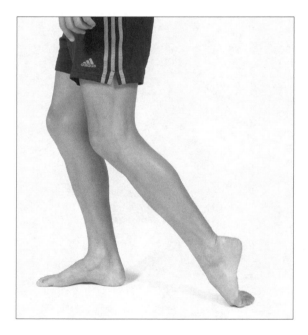

DORSIFLEXORS AND TOE EXTENSORS

1. From a standing position, slide one foot backward and place the top of the foot on the floor with the toes bent under.

2. Bend both knees and lift the ankle of the back foot upward.

3. Gently shift your weight toward back foot.

4. Change the angle of your ankle slightly, turning it inward or outward.

5. To increase the stretch, bend both knees more and shift more weight onto the top of the back foot without compressing the toe joints.

UPPER AND MID BACK

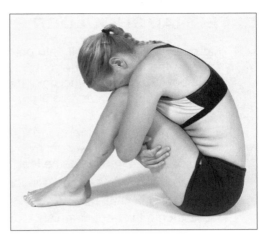

1. Sit on the floor with the legs straight out in front of you. Then bend the knees toward the chest, wrapping the arms around the back of the knees.

2. As you inhale, tuck the chin into the chest, rounding the back away from the thighs. As you exhale, maintain the leg hug, but gently pull the upper back away from the legs while pushing the feet flat into the floor.

3. Gently rock back and forth three times while in this position, then rest in the starting position.

4. Lengthen the spine through the top of the head and lean forward on the toes on inhalation. Curl the spine back down with the chin tucked in when the weight is back on the hips on exhalation.

5. To increase the stretch, rock your weight back into the hips and allow the heels to lift off the floor.

RHOMBOIDS

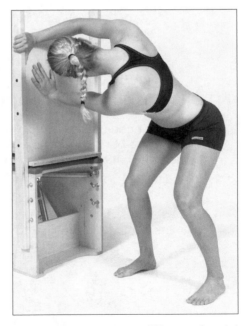

1. Stand in an open doorway (or use a tall stable piece of furniture). Bend forward at the waist and hips at a 90-degree angle and bend both knees. Keep your weight evenly distributed on both legs.

2. Twist your torso toward the doorjamb or piece of furniture and with bottom hand grab the frame on other side of door (or use the flat-hand option pictured).

3. Place the other hand slightly above shoulder height on the same side of the doorjamb or piece of furniture.

4. On exhalation, push away from doorjamb or piece of furniture with the top hand and pull toward the other side with the bottom hand.

5. Explore various hand positions and torso angles to target different fascial fibers.

6. To increase the stretch, position your feet farther away from the doorway or piece of furniture; push slightly harder and pull away more to increase torso rotation.

EXTERNAL SHOULDER ROTATORS

1. Lie on your back and roll onto one side, lying on the shoulder to stabilize it. Position the bottom arm about 60 degrees down from shoulder level. Bend the elbow 90 degrees and point the hand straight up in the air with the palm facing the feet. You can use a pillow or rolled-up towel to support the head if necessary.
2. With the hand of the upper arm, grasp the lower arm above the wrist. Inhale. Then, while exhaling, very gently press the bottom arm and hand down toward the floor in the direction of the feet.
3. Release slowly back to the start position and repeat the stretch as needed.
4. To increase the stretch, move the hand closer to the body or roll the body farther forward onto the front of the shoulder.

The shoulder rotators can be a delicate group of muscles, so take this stretch gently and very slowly.

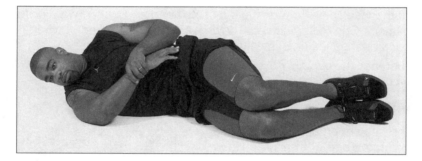

INTERNAL SHOULDER ROTATORS

1. Lie on your back and roll onto one side, lying on the shoulder to stabilize it. The elbow of the bottom arm is bent 90 degrees with the hand pointed straight up in the air with the palm facing upward toward the head.
2. Grasp the bottom wrist with the top hand and slowly, gently press the arm down toward the floor in the direction of the head until you feel a stretch.
3. Release slowly and repeat the stretch as needed, rolling the body farther forward onto the front of the shoulder to increase the stretch.

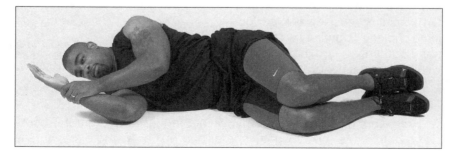

PECTORALIS MAJOR

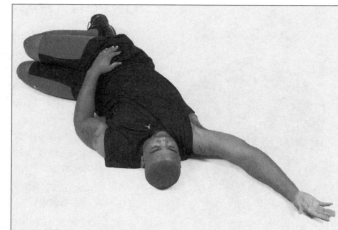

1. Lie on your back and extend one arm out to the side with the palm facing up.

2. As you exhale, bend the knees and drop them to the opposite side of the extended arm.

3. Slowly slide the arm up and down along the floor to target all the pectoral fibers.

4. Repeat on the other side.

5. To increase stretch, reach the hand and arm as far away as possible from the shoulder joint and turn the body away from the arm.

PECTORALIS MINOR

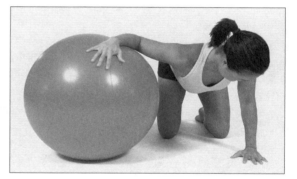

1. Kneel, with one shoulder and elbow at a 90-degree angle. Place the hand and lower arm on a stability ball or other object that is at about shoulder height when kneeling.

2. Place the other hand on the floor directly underneath the shoulder.

3. As you exhale, slowly press the shoulder of the arm on the ball down toward the hand on the floor. Keep the elbow in position on the ball and twist the entire shoulder downward toward the hand on the floor.

4. Release the stretch and repeat.

5. To increase the stretch if using a ball, make very small circles by directing the ball with the shoulder, hand, or both. Or keep the ball still and try various angle changes, moving your torso or rocking back in your hips to feel more variation in the stretch. To increase the stretch, roll the ball forward slightly and drop the shoulder farther downward toward the hand on the floor.

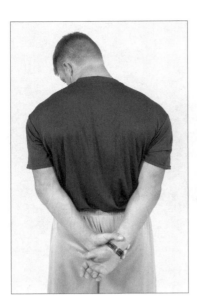

UPPER TRAPEZIUS

1. While standing with one arm held straight and behind the back, grasp the wrist of the arm behind the back with the other hand.
2. Pull the wrist down toward the floor and further behind the body.
3. While holding the wrist, exhale, slowly tilt the head away, opposite from the shoulder of the arm being pulled, and turn the chin downward toward the armpit.
4. Move the head in different directions to target more fibers.
5. To increase the stretch, increase neck flexion to each side and rotation downward and upward, leading with the eyes as you traction the arm farther behind back.

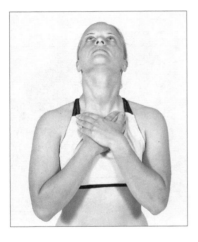

ANTERIOR NECK

1. While sitting upright or standing, cross your arms in front of you and place the hands just above the clavicles.
2. Gently pull down on the front of the neck with hands.
3. Exhale and lift the chin slowly to the ceiling.
4. To increase the stretch, rotate the head into various angles to target more tissue or bend the torso in the same direction as the head while stretching.

LATERAL NECK AND LEVATOR SCAPULA

1. While sitting upright or standing, place one hand on the side of the top of the head.
2. Exhale and slowly bend the neck into lateral flexion; release the stretch on an inhalation and repeat the stretch on an exhalation.
3. To increase the stretch, reach the opposite hand and shoulder down toward the floor.
4. To add a rotation component to this stretch, rotate the head downward so the eyes are looking toward the armpit.
5. Exhale and move the hands back to the top of the head and increase the forward neck bend.
6. To increase the stretch, reach the opposite hand and shoulder down toward the floor.

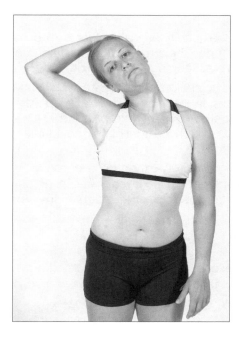 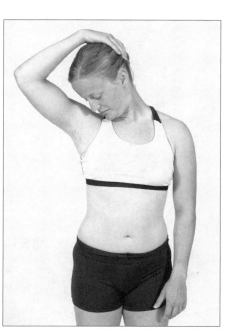

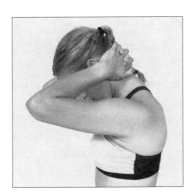

POSTERIOR NECK

1. While standing or sitting upright, interlace the fingers behind the head and inhale as you gently traction the head upward.
2. Exhale and bend head into forward flexion.
3. Bring the elbows together and tuck chin toward chest. Release the stretch and repeat.
4. To increase the stretch, bring elbows closer together.

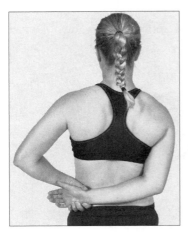

ANTERIOR SHOULDER

1. Relax one shoulder downward and draw that shoulder's arm across the back with other hand.
2. With the hand holding the other arm above the wrist, bring the arm as far across the back as possible, keeping the elbow bent.
3. Stand up straight and exhale as you gently pull the arm farther across the back. To increase the stretch, keep the wrist pressed on the torso as you stretch the front of the shoulder to open it more.
4. To further increase the stretch, continue pulling the arm behind the low back as far across the back as possible, and straighten the elbow.

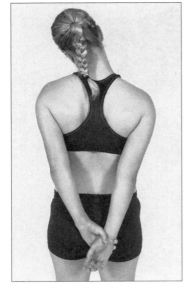

MEDIAL SHOULDER

1. Relax one shoulder downward and draw that shoulder's arm across the back with other hand.
2. With the hand holding the other arm above the wrist, pull the arm downward toward the floor and opposite leg, keeping the elbow straight.
3. To increase the stretch, exhale as you bend the head into lateral flexion to the opposite side of the shoulder being stretched.

POSTERIOR SHOULDER

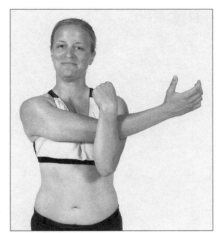

1. Relax one shoulder downward and draw that shoulder's arm across your chest with other hand. Slide the bottom arm that is assisting under the arm being stretched, and cross the elbows.
2. Bring the arm being stretched toward the body and as far across the chest as possible, keeping the elbow straight by bending the assisting arm more.
3. Exhale as you gently pull the arm across chest, making sure the shoulder stays dropped downward.
4. To increase the stretch, you can change the position of the assisting arm to hold the arm being stretched above the wrist. Then internally rotate the arm and traction it away from the body.

BICEPS

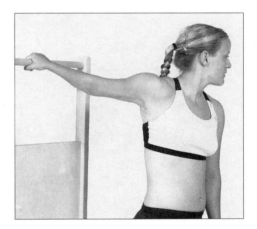

1. Grasp a pole or doorjamb with one hand at shoulder height.
2. Turn the hand with the thumb pointing downward.
3. Try to rotate the entire arm down toward floor.
4. To increase the stretch, twist the torso away from the arm, exhaling into the stretch.

TRICEPS

1. From a kneeling position, place the elbows and the forearms on a stable object.
2. Bend the elbows and grasp one wrist with the other hand, holding it behind the head. Exhale and bend the elbow of the grasped arm even more.
3. To increase the stretch, press the wrist and fingertips farther toward the back or press the lower torso toward the floor on an exhalation. Repeat on the other side.

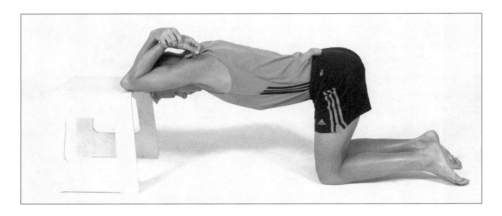

FOREARM AND WRIST EXTENSORS

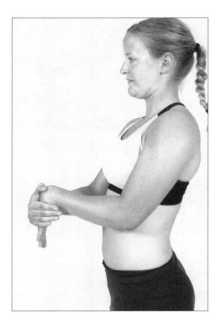

1. Gently traction, or pull out, one of your wrists by grasping the hand of that wrist with the other hand.
2. Exhale, bend the wrist into flexion, and place the assisting hand over the top of the wrist being stretched.
3. Relax the elbow and shoulder downward as you bend the fingertips toward the body.
4. To increase the stretch, slide the assisting hand down to the fingertips and straighten the elbow.
5. Explore different angles by moving the hand in different directions.
6. Finish the stretch by pulling the wrist again. Repeat on the other side.

FOREARM AND WRIST FLEXORS

1. Traction one of your wrists by grasping the hand with the other hand and pulling gently.
2. As you exhale, bend the wrist into extension and place the assisting hand palm to palm with the wrist being stretched.
3. Relax the elbow and shoulder as you bend the fingers toward the body, making sure to include the thumb.
4. To increase the stretch, slide the assisting hand down to the fingertips and straighten the elbow.
5. Explore different angles by moving the hand in different directions.
6. Traction the wrist again to finish the stretch. Repeat sequence on the other side.

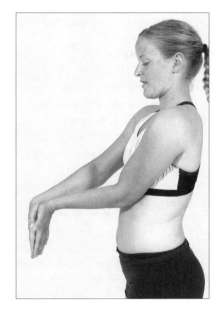

HAND

1. Press the palms together and spread the fingers apart.
2. Open the elbows out to the sides, keeping the shoulders down.
3. Exhale and drop the wrists downward as you press the palms and fingertips together.
4. Raise the elbows out to the sides, separating the wrists while gently continuing to press only the fingertips together.
5. Roll the fingers and palms back together, pressing gently.
6. To increase stretch, continue lifting the elbows away from the body.

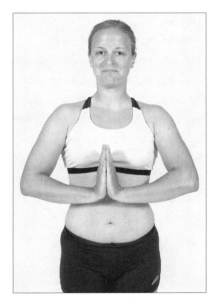

Restorative Stretches

These are good stretches to do at the end of the day or to put together as a restorative routine anytime. They cover all areas of the body, focusing particularly on the hip area, which, as we discuss early in this chapter, often needs the most attention. Some of the stretches in this program are made up of some of the key stretches linked together in a series. The idea is that you flow from one stretch right into the next one. The transitional movements should be done during inhalations and the stretches should be done during exhalations.

Full Restorative Program

While the restorative stretches are presented in the basic order of our full restorative program, our program also uses some of the key stretches described on pages 126 to 145. For the full description of each key stretch used in this program, see the indicated page number in the list that follows. This routine has been designed to allow you to move easily from one stretch into the next with a smooth flow and rhythm. You may choose to do only a few of the sequences in this routine. You can also add other stretches for your specific needs. Again, the concept is to be able to customize your program and change it as needed.

1. Hip warm-up, page 149
2. Hip openers, page 149
3. Front of hip and torso series, pages 150-151
4. Gluteus complex (see core four, page 125)
5. Quadratus lumborum and latissimus dorsi (see core four, page 126)
6. Low back series, pages 152-153
7. Lying gluteus maximus and medius (see key stretches, page 129)
8. Hamstring series, pages 154-156
9. Arm series, pages 157-159
10. Hip flexor series, pages 160-161
11. Full fascial stretch, pages 162-163

HIP WARM-UP

Although this movement warms up the entire hip region, it focuses on the lateral aspect of the hip and the joint capsule.

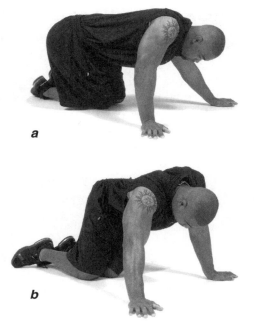

a

1. Start on your hands and knees, with your hands placed wider than the shoulders, fingers pointing outward, and knees together.
2. Exhale and slowly rock hips to the right side.
3. Inhale as you slowly return them back to center.
4. Exhale and slowly rock hips to the left side.
5. Continue rocking side to side, moving slightly farther out each time, until you feel that you have loosened up considerably and that the movement is freer.

b

HIP OPENERS

This movement focuses on the rotational components of the hip.

1. Sit on the ground with the knees bent and the feet slightly wider than hip-width apart, feet flat on the floor. Place the arms behind you with palms on the floor and fingers pointing away from the body.
2. Exhale, lean the torso back, and slowly drop both knees to the right side.
3. Inhale and return to center. Then exhale and repeat, dropping both knees to the left.
4. Continue dropping the knees side to side, visualizing them as a wave, until both legs can touch the floor or you feel considerably looser.

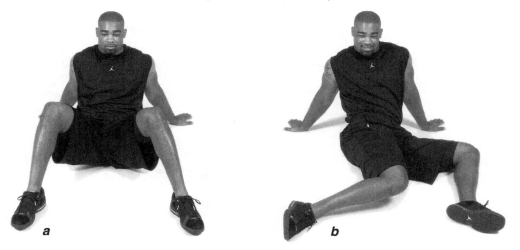

a   *b*

FRONT OF HIP AND TORSO SERIES

During this series, think of yourself as waving up into the stretch and waving back down to the floor.

1. Start on your hands and knees. Lower your upper body toward the ground, placing your hands beneath your shoulders as if you were doing a push-up.

2. Inhale, then press your hands into the floor, exhaling as you lift your upper body up as far as possible without allowing any pinching in the low back. Keep the pelvis, knees, and toes down and relaxed. Keep hips pressing toward the ground and lengthen the spine through the top of the head.

3. Inhale and release the stretch, then exhale and sit back on the heels.

4. Inhale to return to the stretch position, and repeat the sequence back and forth until tension in the tissue is greatly reduced.

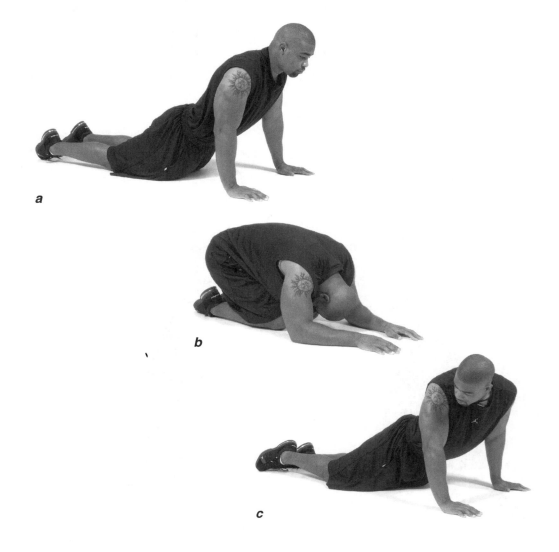

a

b

c

5. Now, from the lifted stretch position, rotate the torso to one side and exhale while pressing weight into the opposite hand.

6. Inhale and return to the center position.

7. Repeat the torso rotation to the other side, and continue moving side to side until you feel loose. You may increase the stretch by lifting your chin to the ceiling to finish the last stretch.

8. Sit back onto the heels with the upper body on the ground to relax the body and release any tension that you may have felt in the low back during the stretch series.

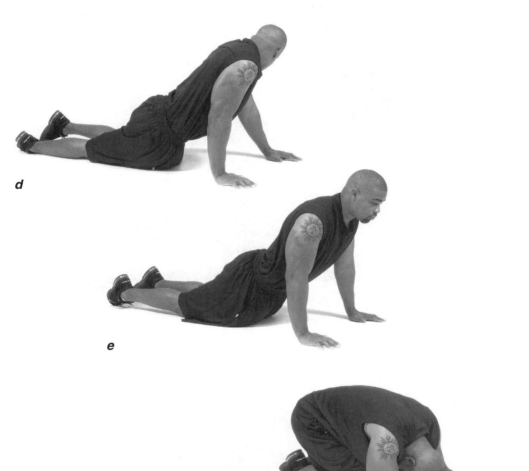

d

e

f

LOW BACK SERIES

This series targets the low back and the lateral hips.

1. Inhale, then pull both knees into your chest with your hands as you exhale. Repeat with increasing range.

2. Drop the arms out to side and drop both legs to one side with an exhalation. Lift them to the center as you inhale and drop them to the other side as you exhale, repeating as necessary until you feel loose.

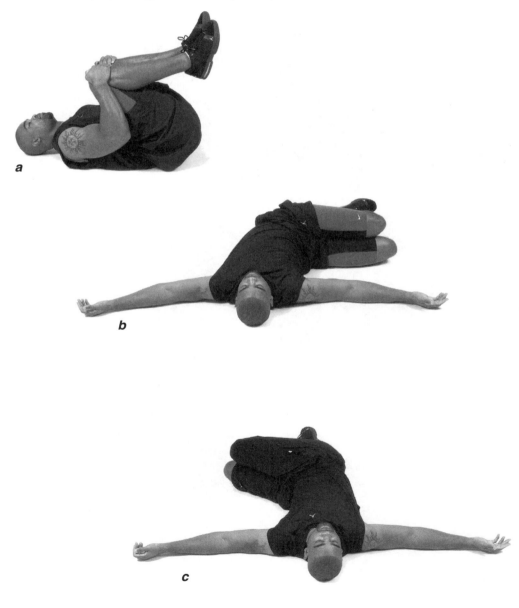

a

b

c

3. From the position of the knees dropped to one side, slide the top leg over the bottom leg and allow the top leg to touch the floor. Inhale. On an exhalation press the top knee down toward the floor with the hand. Release the hand pressure as you inhale, then press the knee down again as you exhale, repeating the sequence as necessary.

4. To increase the stretch, slide the bottom leg backward as far away from the top leg as possible and press the knee to the floor, keeping both shoulders on the floor. To further increase the stretch, reach the free arm overhead.

5. Repeat series on other side.

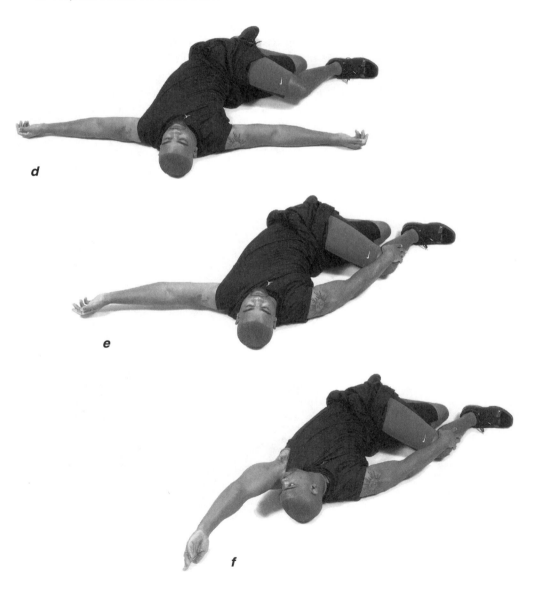

d

e

f

HAMSTRING SERIES

Athletes probably stretch the hamstrings more than any other group of muscles, but they seldom target all the angles and fibers that maximize flexibility in this crucial area.

1. First stretch the gluteus maximus and deep rotators and the gluteus medius (page 129).

2. Lie on your back, relaxed. Bend the knee of one leg, placing the foot on the floor. Bend the knee of the other leg, placing the foot on floor. Interlace the fingertips behind the bent knee.

3. Keeping the head and shoulders relaxed on the floor, inhale, then exhale as you gently stretch one bent leg upward and outward from the joint and then toward center of chest. To increase the stretch, try to bring the leg closer to the chest with each exhalation.

4. Inhale, then gently stretch the leg up and outward from the joint and toward the shoulder on the same side. To increase the stretch, try to bring the leg closer to the shoulder with each exhalation.

5. Inhale, then exhale as you take the lifted leg across the body and up toward the opposite shoulder. Gently stretch the leg upward and outward from the joint toward the opposite shoulder. To increase the stretch, try to bring the leg farther across the chest with each exhalation.

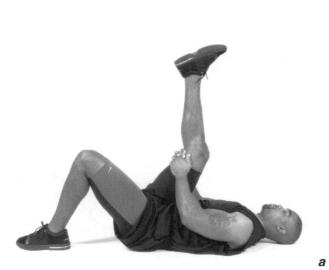 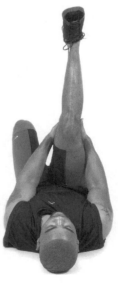

a

6. Bring the leg back to center. Inhale, then exhale as you straighten the knee while you pull the toes toward the chest until you feel the stretch.

7. Inhale and release the stretch. Repeat as needed.

8. Bring the leg to the same-side shoulder and straighten the knee, then bring the leg over to the opposite shoulder and straighten the knee.

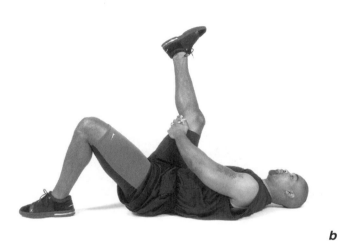

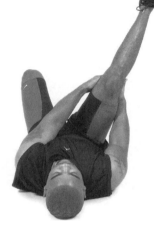

b

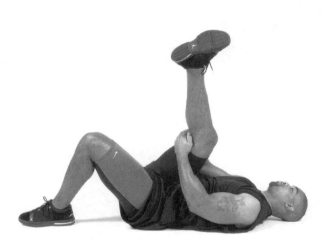

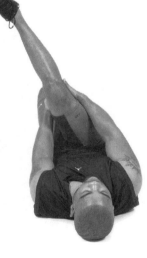

c

(continued)

(continued)

9. Bring the leg back to the center and flex the foot. To intensify the stretch, inhale, then exhale as you raise your head, performing an abdominal crunch in the stretch position. Inhale as you return the head to the floor and relax the stretch. Repeat as needed.

10. Lower the stretching leg down to the floor in front of you and sit up. Keep the opposite leg bent behind you. Lean the torso over to the outside of the stretched leg, supporting yourself with the hands on the floor.

11. Using the stretch wave motion, inhale and raise the torso up to the top of the head, then lower it as you exhale. To repeat, raise the torso up again as you inhale, then lower as you exhale, reaching the torso out and down even farther as your body allows. Repeat as needed.

12. To increase the stretch, flex and internally rotate the foot of the leg being stretched.

13. Roll back onto the back and repeat the series on the other side.

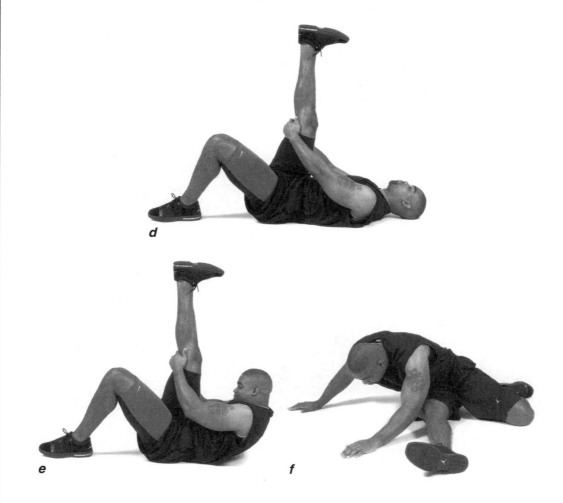

d

e   *f*

ARM SERIES

This series targets the external and internal rotator muscles of the shoulder, as well as the pectorals, biceps, triceps, posterior and middle deltoids, and the rhomboids.

1. Lie on your back and roll onto one side, lying on the shoulder to stabilize it. You may use a pillow or rolled-up towel to support the head. Position the bottom arm about 45 degrees down from shoulder level. Bend the elbow 90 degrees and point the hand straight up in the air with the palm facing the feet.

2. With the hand of the upper arm, grasp the lower arm above the wrist. Inhale. Then, while exhaling, very gently press the bottom arm and palm down toward the floor in the direction of the feet.

3. Release slowly back to the start position and repeat the stretch as needed. To increase the stretch, move the hand closer to the body or roll the body farther up onto the shoulder.

4. Now position the bottom arm about 90 degrees down from shoulder level. Bend the elbow 90 degrees and point the hand straight up in the air with the palm facing the ceiling.

5. Place the top hand on the other arm and grasp the wrist. Slowly and gently press the arm down toward the floor in the direction of the head until you feel a stretch.

6. Release slowly and repeat the stretch as needed, rolling the body farther onto the shoulder to increase the stretch.

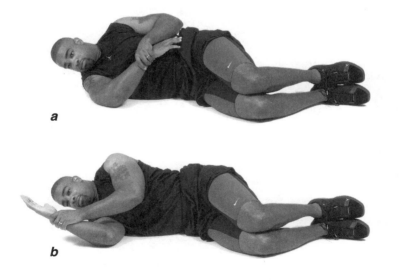

a

b

(continued)

(continued)

7. Bring both legs out in front of you, bend the knees, and then lie on your back, arms down by your sides.

8. Inhale, then drop the knees to one side.

9. Exhale as you slowly slide the arm on the other side of the knees along the floor toward the head. You should feel the different fibers of the shoulder and chest stretch as you change the angle of the arm. Continue sliding the arm until you either touch your head or feel the movement stop.

10. Inhale, then exhale as you return the arm back to your side. Repeat this sequence as needed. To increase the stretch, reach out of the shoulder socket as you move the arm along the path of the stretch. If you feel a pinching sensation in the shoulder, return the arm to your side and repeat with less effort or reach.

11. Return the arm out from the side and internally rotate the arm and hand as you turn the head away from the outstretched arm. To intensify the stretch, increase the internal rotation of the thumb.

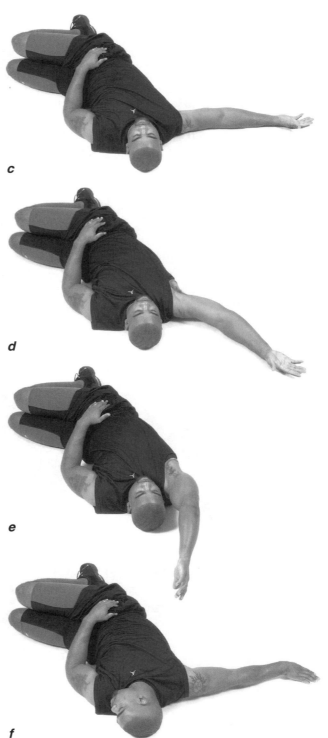

c

d

e

f

12. Straighten the legs and roll onto the belly with the arms extended straight in front of you.

13. Inhale, then exhale as you bend the elbow of the shoulder just stretched, helping it by grasping the wrist with the other hand until you feel a stretch in the triceps. If tight, you may also feel it in the lats. Make sure that you let the head and back relax as you stretch. To increase the stretch, press the wrist and fingertips down toward the back as you press the armpit into the floor.

14. Straighten out the arm that was just stretched, and with the other hand push into the floor to roll the body back onto the side.

15. Slide the outstretched arm down along the floor until it is across the chest. Exhale and slowly roll the body back to the stomach with the outstretched arm underneath. Reach the top arm over the other arm and place it on the floor.

16. Inhale, then exhale as you roll the body back toward the shoulder.

17. Reach the arm being stretched farther from the body and roll the body back over the arm until you feel a stretch anywhere from the back of the shoulder joint to the area between the shoulder blades. Inhale as you slowly roll slightly off the arm to ease off the stretch. Repeat as needed. To increase the stretch, press the palm into the floor and lift the shoulder slightly off the floor.

18. Roll off your arm and onto your side, then onto all fours to *slowly* stand up. If you feel dizzy, go back down to all fours and take several deep breaths before attempting to stand again.

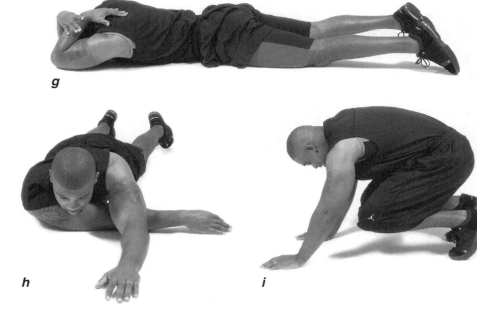

g

h

i

HIP FLEXOR SERIES

This series targets the muscles of the hip flexors, lateral hip, and groin.

1. From standing, kneel in a lunge position with the right leg back. Inhale, keeping the chest lifted and abdominal muscles pulled slightly inward.

2. Exhale, pressing the right hip forward until you feel a slight stretch. Inhale and release the stretch and your body slightly. Then wave into the stretch on the exhalation again. Repeat the stretch wave as many times as necessary, using the breathing pattern just described, until you feel the tissue release.

3. To progress the stretch along the front fascial line, inhale and reach the right arm upward, then exhale, lunging into the stretch wave and maintaining a lifted torso and slightly arched back. Drop your arm and inhale as you release the stretch and return to start position.

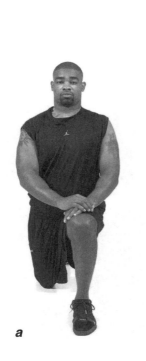
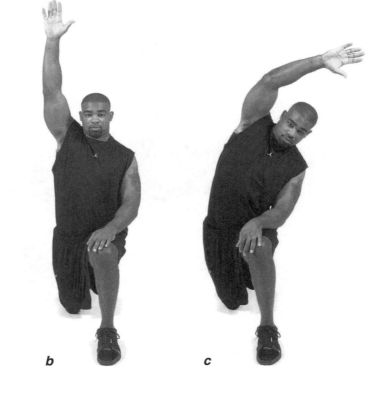

a   *b*   *c*

4. To continue the stretch into the lateral line of the hips and torso, inhale and lean the body over to the left side and push the right hip slightly outward as you exhale into stretch. Inhale as you release.

5. From the leaning position, rotate the torso by turning the chest upward. Reach the right hand upward and turn the palm to the ceiling. Experiment with the angles of your arm as you exhale. Repeat until you feel all the tissues are moving freely.

6. Inhale, then exhale as you lean the torso away from the back leg, simultaneously gently pushing the hip of the back leg to the outside until you feel a gentle stretch. Repeat as needed.

7. Inhale, then exhale and step the front leg out to a side lunge until you feel a stretch. Inhale and reduce the lunge to decrease the stretch. To increase the stretch, deepen the lunge. Repeat as needed, then stretch the other side.

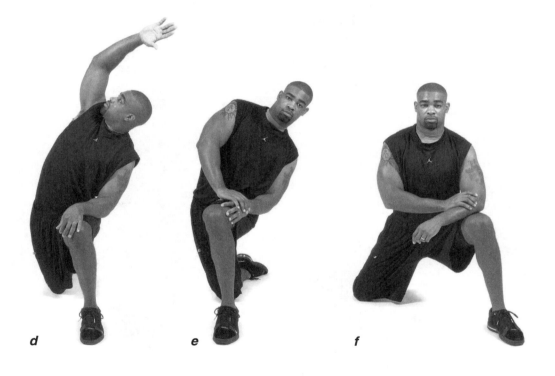

d e f

FULL FASCIAL STRETCH

We recommend finishing with a stretch of all the main fascial lines. The sequence should flow smoothly

1. Move into an all fours position and slowly roll the body up to a standing position; this is called a back line roll up.

2. From a standing position, inhale and reach the head, arms, and torso up. Exhale and bend slightly backward.

3. Bend the knees slightly as you return to the standing position with the arms down by your side. Repeat as needed.

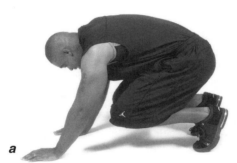

a

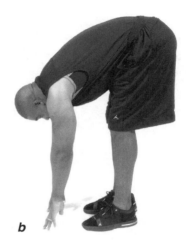

b

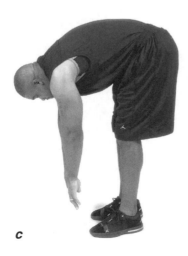

c

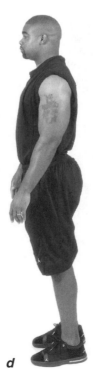

d

e

4. Inhale, then exhale as you raise one arm up and reach the head and torso up; then lean over to the opposite side of the raised arm until you feel the stretch. Continue the movement forward until you are bent over forward at the waist before coming up to repeat on the other side.

5. Reach up with head, arms, and torso and then gently lean back to finish the series.

f

g

Stretches Using Props

Several of the key stretches on pages 127 to 147 take advantage of balls, walls, poles, bands, and other objects for outside leverage. Sometimes such tools offer the best way to stretch an area. They can help you improve your flexibility even more by providing resistance for self-proprioceptive neuromuscular facilitation (PNF), increasing the efficiency of this powerful technique.

As you'll remember from principle 9 in chapter 1 (page 14), facilitating body reflexes through a method such as PNF or assisted stretching with a partner helps you to reach optimal flexibility. Research has proven that PNF yields the greatest gains in ROM in the shortest amount of time. It has also shown that gains in ROM resulting from PNF contract-release (CR) stretching lasted the longest over time when compared to other stretching techniques.

While you can use PNF in many of the stretches in our system, it is most effective with those in which you use an object or prop. In chapter 8, we discuss specific ways to use PNF techniques with partner-assisted stretching.

Among the many props you can use to add variety to your stretching routine are the following:

- **Stability balls.** Stability or physio balls are one of our favorite choices for stretching props because of their three-dimensional quality and pliability. Choose a ball between 45 and 75 centimeters in diameter—the taller the person, the larger the diameter of the ball should be. If you desire more stability when using a ball, rest one side of the ball against a wall for any of the stretches. In addition to the adductor ball stretch we use the ball in the key stretches for the hip flexors (page 130), quadriceps (page 132), quadratus lumborum and iliotibial band (page 130), and pectoralis minor (page 141).

- **Walls, doorways, and stable objects.** Using a wall or doorjamb is great when you need an unmovable object for stability. For our photos we substituted a Pilates chair for the wall (often a piece of stable furniture or equipment works for wall stretches). The lateral line wall stretch on page 166 targets the lateral line, including the QL, ITB, obliques, and latissimus dorsi.

- **Chairs and benches.** A chair or bench is a good object to help you stretch, especially when you want to be up off the ground and don't want to be concerned about keeping your balance. We suggest using a chair or a bench that is stable and that allows you to place your feet flat on the floor with the knees bent at 90 degrees.

- **Bands, ropes, and towels.** We find that using bands, ropes, or towels in stretching is beneficial when you need more leverage. If you have short arms in relation to your legs or if you are very tight (we refer to it as "flexibility challenged"), they can be especially helpful. When choosing a Theraband, choose one that is at least medium weight for strength. Bands, ropes and towels should be long enough to wrap around the ball of the foot while holding each end comfortably in each hand.

ADDUCTOR BALL STRETCH

1. Sit just in front of the top of the ball with legs apart and both knees bent 90 degrees with the feet flat on the floor.
2. Shift your weight onto one leg and straighten the other leg as much as possible, while keeping the ball of the foot on the floor for balance.
3. Bend over from the waist as you exhale.
4. To increase the stretch, bring the elbow on the same side as the extended leg toward the bent leg and continue to straighten the extended leg. You can change the feel of the stretch by exploring different positions on the ball.

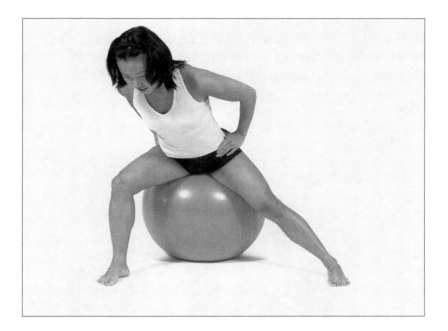

LATERAL LINE WALL STRETCH

1. Stand about 2 feet (61 cm) from the wall or stable surface with your side facing it. With feet together, place the hand closest to the wall or surface on it. Put the other hand on the hip and inhale.

2. Exhale as you lean your hips into the surface.

3. To increase the stretch, lean the upper body away from the surface as you continue pressing the hips toward the wall.

4. Now turn to face the surface with your feet 2 feet (61 cm) from the wall and hip-width apart.

5. Lean your body toward the surface, placing both hands on it, one above the other. Inhale.

6. Exhale as you push against the surface with the hands. To increase the stretch, straighten your arms and continue pushing away.

7. Now bring the feet together and inhale.

8. Exhale as you rotate the chest toward the top arm and ceiling and bend laterally toward the surface, slightly arching your back.

9. To increase the stretch, continue rotating the torso until the top arm comes off the surface.

10. To further increase the stretch, touch the wall with fingertips, completely rotating the chest upward toward the top arm.

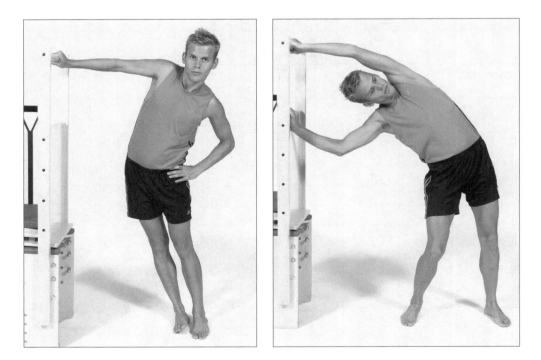

LOW BACK CHAIR STRETCH

1. Sit on a chair or bench and open each leg out to the side with the knees bent and feet flat on the floor. Inhale.

2. Exhale and round the torso over toward the floor, relaxing the upper body and head.

3. Reach through the legs with the arms and continue lowering the upper body and head to the floor, using the breathing pattern just described.

4. Move the torso to the right and reach both arms through the right leg, using the recommended breathing pattern. Repeat on the left side.

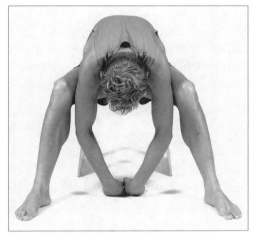

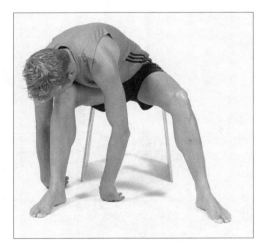

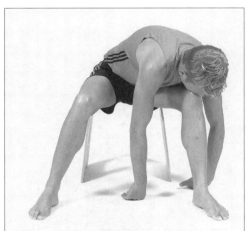

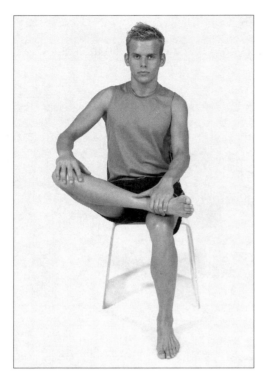

GLUTE CHAIR STRETCH

1. Sit upright in a chair with the feet flat on the ground. Cross one leg over the other so that the ankle rests above the knee. Inhale.

2. Exhale. Press the knee gently down toward the floor with the hand belonging to same side as the leg; hold the ankle in place with the other hand.

3. Lean forward with the torso and continue pressing the knee toward the floor.

4. Turn the torso away from the crossed leg and continue pressing the knee toward the floor.

5. To increase the stretch, bring the shoulder of the crossed leg toward the lifted foot.

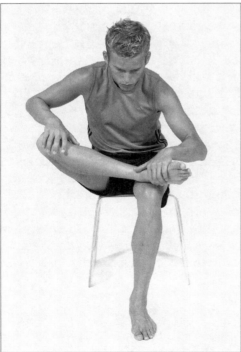

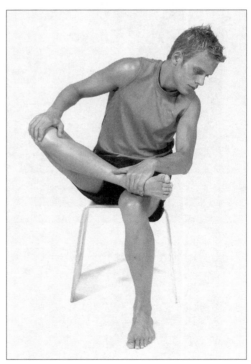

HIP FLEXOR
CHAIR STRETCH

1. Stand facing a chair or bench, bend one knee and place the same-side foot on the seat. Square the hips and inhale.

2. Exhale. Lift the torso up and press both hips forward, especially from the leg on the floor.

3. Move in and out of this stretch until you feel a release in the resistance of the hip flexors.

4. To increase the stretch, lift the torso upward and arch the back into extension, being careful not to pinch the low back. Continue pressing both hips forward.

5. To further increase stretch, lift the arm opposite the bent leg up over the head while in back extension and then lift up the other arm.

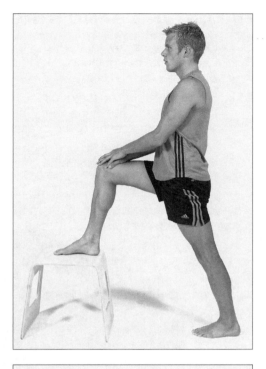

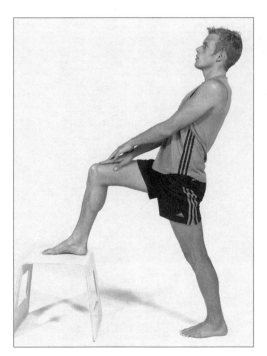

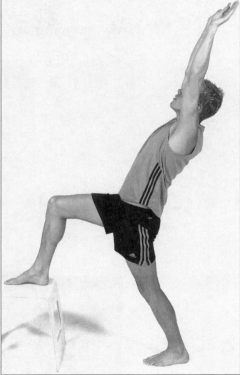

HAMSTRING BAND STRETCH

1. Lie on your back with one leg straight. Slightly bend the other leg and place a band on the ball of the foot, keeping the foot relaxed. Let the head and shoulders relax on the floor.
2. Focus on stretching the origin of the hamstrings first. To do this, gently stretch the leg up and out of the joint, bending the knee slightly, and then stretch the leg toward the center of the chest.
3. To increase the stretch, with each exhalation try to bring leg closer to the chest; to further increase the stretch, straighten the knee.

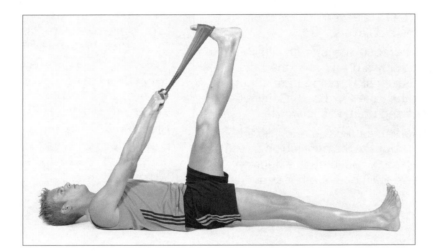

4. Now open the leg out to the side. Keep the knee slightly bent as you focus on stretching the origin of the hamstring.

5. Gently stretch the leg up and outward from the joint and down toward the floor.

6. To increase this part of the stretch, with each exhalation try to bring the leg closer to the shoulder on the same side and toward the floor, as well as straightening the knee.

7. Now take the leg across the body toward the floor on the opposite side. Keep the knee slightly bent again.

8. Gently stretch the leg up and outward from the joint toward the center of the chest.

9. To increase the stretch, with each exhalation try to bring the leg closer, across the chest and toward the opposite shoulder, as well as straightening the knee.

Begin with a slightly bent knee for all positions and then straighten knee if possible. Use the band to help traction the leg up in the hip socket and guide the leg to each side.

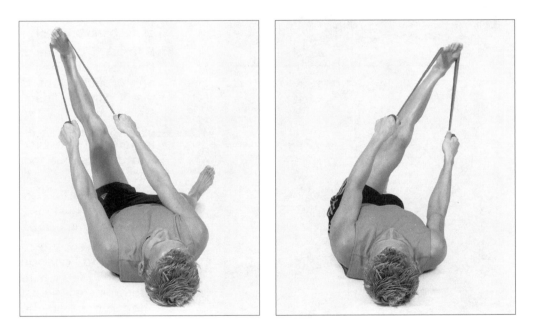

SOLEUS AND GASTROCNEMIUS BAND STRETCH

1. Sit on the floor. Extend one leg in front of you and bend the other leg with the foot flat on the floor.
2. Wrap a band, rope, or towel around the ball of the foot of the bent leg.

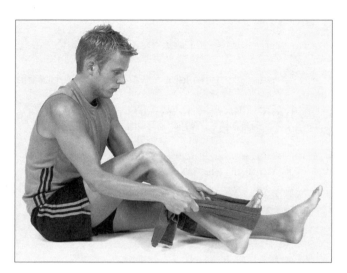

3. Sit up tall with the torso and dorsiflex the foot back toward your body, using the band or towel to assist. Inhale and gently push the ball of the foot into the band for three to six seconds with about 50 percent of your strength against the resistance of the band.

4. Exhale and increase dorsiflexion with the aid of the band or towel.

5. Repeat a couple of times and change the angle of the foot to target different fibers. Or, to increase the stretch, you can lean forward with the torso and dorsiflex the foot back farther.

6. Now straighten the bent leg and repeat steps 2 to 5 on the same leg.

7. Repeat a couple of times and change angle of the foot to target different fibers. Then repeat on the other side.

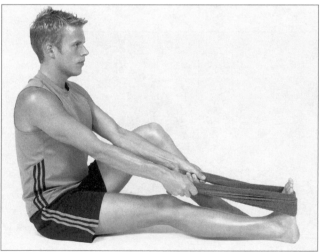

Stretching in a Heated Environment

Some of the best places to do recovery and maintenance stretching are in the steam room, sauna, whirlpool, bathtub, and shower. Naturally, the heated environment is one of the main appeals—heat stimulates blood flow and perspiration for elimination of toxins, and it also increases the viscoelasticity of the connective tissues, which relaxes the body and improves its response to stretching. All of this decreases myofascial tension and tone and encourages the athlete to enter the state in which the parasympathetic nervous system is dominant.

One of the few things that experts in this field agree on is the importance of raising the body's core temperature for safer stretching. Research clearly shows that even warming the body passively, such as by soaking in a warm bath, increases many favorable conditions for maximizing flexibility. This can also solve one of the most common problems of athletes who want to develop their flexibility: lack of time. A heated setting is excellent for recovering from the stress and strain of intensive athletic work.

You obtain the best results for this warm-body stretching within the hour before you go to sleep; slip into a very warm tub (as warm as tolerated) to help unwind the tension that has accumulated over the course of the day. After relaxing by submerging the entire body up to the neck in the tub for at least 10 but no more than 15 minutes or by taking a very warm shower for 10 to 15 minutes come out of the tub or shower and stretch the areas of the body that have been particularly stressed that day. You can usually sense what has become tight or sore within an hour of cooling down from training or competing. Listen to your body and give it what it is asking for at this special time of the day. How you use this time will determine the outcome of performance the next day. By stretching at this time, you can regain flexibility, avoid tightening up overnight, and help prevent the soreness and tightness that most athletes feel the morning after hard training or competition. Hopefully, you will reduce your need to rely on painkillers, anti-inflammatories, or an excessive intake of energy drinks by following this regimen. The results will occur after the first week of trying this routine and will get better and better if you keep the routine going.

Another option is to stretch while in the steam room, sauna, or whirlpool, but again, for no more than 15 minutes at a time. If you stay in the heated environment longer than that, the natural tendency of the body to fluctuate will start having negative effects as the body attempts to regulate its physiology and cool itself off. If you find you require more stretching after the 10 to 15 minutes, cool off for a few minutes in a cool shower, then return to the heated environment and resume stretching after your body has warmed up sufficiently for another set of 10 minutes.

The special setting of the sauna or steam room requires that you use a rolled-up towel as a prop to support bony parts of the leg that are set on the room's steps and sitting benches. It will also protect your foot or leg from the hot surface while you are stretching. If you are sitting in a whirlpool, you will have to improvise, since the buoyancy effect of the water will take over. For many people, the water's tendency to lift the leg or torso is helpful when stretching, but it does require a little more stability and control until you get used to it. You have to be creative and try a range of stretches in a variety of heated settings to find what is convenient and works best for you.

Stretching the Myofascial Lines

A perfect way to complete any stretch routine is do full body myofascial line stretching. There are four basic lines: the front, or anterior, line; the back, or posterior, line; the side, or lateral, line; and the inside, or deep front, line. These lines are also touched on to some degree in chapter 5 relative to self-myofascial release (pages 99 to 102). It is important to understand the value of incorporating all the fascial components, including these lines, to maximize your flexibility potential. Imagine stretching these lines from your fingertips to your toes in the direction of the line in order to truly experience the stretch.

Remember from chapter 2 that myofascia is fascia that wraps around and in between muscles and their fibers and that connects to joints. Including as much fascia as possible when stretching is where most of the potential for increased flexibility exists, so it is important to understand how to stretch fascia using the fascial lines as a guide. You can begin with the lines we've mentioned and then go on to explore the many other lines of fascial connections and stretching directions.

Extending the stretch all the way to the ends of the fascial lines can truly maximize your flexibility. Remember that the fascia goes in many directions and has many layers. This is where you'll find that by changing your position ever so slightly you can find new areas of tightness. These stretches can tell you how much room for improvement there is in your body. Explore the different lines and see what needs the most attention.

> When I began doing my nighttime stretch routine regularly, I felt an immediate impact on how good and loose my body felt in the morning and throughout my day.
>
> *Jeremiah Trotter,*
> *Three-Time*
> *NFL Pro Bowler*

The following is a condensed list of the main fascial lines and the main myofascial groups directly associated with them, starting at the foot and ending at the head (adapted from Myers 2001):

Front line—toe extensor muscles, tibialis anterior and anterior leg fascia, quadriceps, iliacus and psoas muscles, rectus abdominis, sternalis and sternochondral fascia, sternocleidomastoid, scalp fascia

Back line—toe flexor muscles, plantar fascia, Achilles tendon and gastrocnemius-soleus, hamstrings, sacrotuberous and sacrolumbar fascia, erector spinae, scalp fascia

Lateral line—peroneal muscles and lateral leg fascia, iliotibial tract, tensor fascia latae, hip abductor muscles, gluteus maximus, lateral abdominal obliques, external and internal intercostals, sternocleidomastoid and splenius capitis muscles, shoulder abductors

Deep front line–posterior tibialis tendon and the fascia of the inside leg, hip adductors, shoulder adductors

FRONT LINE

1. Stand with the feet hip-width or more apart.
2. Reach the hands up over the head.
3. Slowly inhale as you lift the torso up and bend the back into extension.
4. Continue to slowly inhale as you stretch the body all the way through the fingertips and bend back as far as possible. You should feel the stretch through the front of your body.
5. Exhale and release back to standing upright.
6. To increase the stretch, flex the hands back and lift the chin to the ceiling in back extension.

BACK LINE

1. Stand with the feet hip-distance apart. Bend at the hips and put the hands on the floor; inhale and walk them away from the feet.
2. Keep the heels down and press the palms into the floor.
3. Bend the knees if necessary; attempt to straighten them as you continue stretching.
4. Exhale and push the torso down toward the floor and the hips back toward your heels. You should feel the stretch in the back of the body.
5. To increase the stretch, walk the hands back to the feet as you inhale.
6. Exhale and hug the arms around the back of the knees.
7. To increase the stretch farther, shift your weight slightly forward and pull the torso closer to the legs.

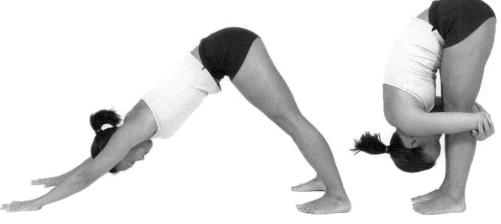

SIDE LINE

1. With feet slightly apart, place one arm on the side of the upper leg. Inhale and reach the other arm up over the head.

2. Slowly inhale and bend toward the side with the arm on the leg.

3. Stretch through the fingertips and bend as far as possible. You should feel this stretch on the side of the body you are bending away from.

4. Explore different angles by gently rotating the torso.

5. To increase the stretch, turn the top arm so the palm faces upward.

6. Exhale as you return to the start, then repeat on the other side.

DEEP FRONT LINE

1. Stand with the feet as far apart as comfortable. Turn the feet outward into external rotation as much as comfortably possible.

2. Inhale and reach the hands up over the head.

3. Exhale as you lift the torso up and bend the back into extension.

4. Stretch the body all the way through the fingertips and bend back as far as possible. You should feel this stretch deep inside the front of your body.

5. Release back to standing upright.

6. To increase the stretch, open the arms farther apart, and flex the hands and fingertips as far backward as possible. Lift the chin to the ceiling in back extension.

Tips for Stretching the Main Fascial Lines

- Visualize feeling longer or taller before you go into the stretch.
- Initiate movement of the fascia either from the head or the feet.
- Move the fascia from the center of the body or from the end farthest from your center.
- Fascia will stretch most when the two farthest ends of the fascial line move away from each other. This can only be safely accomplished by preparing the body beforehand through either a proper warm-up that heats up the body or through self-myofascial release.

Now that we have shown all the basic stretches in the Stretch to Win matrix, let's take a look at the sport application of these stretches and others in the next chapter.

chapter 7

Sport-Specific Stretches

Athletes use many different kinds of movements in their sports: running, kicking, throwing, hitting, jumping, cutting, swinging, sliding, squatting, twisting, reaching, bending, pivoting, rotating, accelerating, decelerating, changing directions, stopping, starting, unilateral movements, bilateral movements, repetitive movements, and any combination of these actions. In any given sport, the body can perform countless motions and move in countless directions. Have you ever really thought about what kinds of movements are involved in your sport and are necessary to excel in it? Have you ever thought about what movements you do that may not be as smooth or easy to execute as they could be? Or have you ever considered that you might need to unwind by stretching in opposite directions and patterns from those that you use in your sport?

When athletes come to our clinic for a first visit, we usually give them only two or three key stretches to work on initially. There are two main reasons for this. First, when they do only a couple of stretches that target just those areas that have the most restrictions (usually in the hip region), our clients achieve greater results in terms of overall increases in functional athletic movement than they would achieve by doing a lot of stretches designed for other areas. Second, our clinical experience has shown

179

repeatedly that athletes are more compliant and actually do the stretches faithfully if we only give them two or three to do. We teach them a few of the core stretches and begin setting the foundation for them to build their own matrix. We often take digital photos of them doing the stretches and print these out for them to take home. They rarely believe that these couple of stretches can have much effect, but they promise to do them nonetheless. When they return in a few days' or weeks' time, they are amazed at how well the stretches have worked.

Once our clients understand how doing some of the right stretches can improve their flexibility, they become excited about developing a more extensive program to maximize their flexibility potential. They gain a sense of hope and accomplishment from their newfound flexibility. They often report that after doing just the couple of key stretches before bed, they no longer wake up stiff in the morning. Or, if they do their stretches right before a workout or practice, they notice more freedom of movement throughout the activity. These gains are very encouraging.

As you learned in chapter 6, the basic concept of developing your own matrix is to begin with a couple of core stretches that are the most needed and build your program from there. You can create your own custom program that changes as your goals and needs change. The type of program can vary significantly between what you need in-season and perhaps a more extensive program for when you are out of season and have more time and the chance to make real progress with your flexibility. After you consider what muscle groups and movement patterns you use most in your sport and training, you can decide what should take priority in your program.

Building a Flexibility Reserve

When our athletes achieve about 20 percent more ROM in their trunk, spine, shoulders, pelvis, and hips than is required in their sport, they gain what we refer to as a *reserve* of flexibility. We see a significant decrease in injuries in athletes who have this cushion. The reserve comes into use, for example, when an athlete goes down from a hit during a football game and lands in a position that would normally strain or tear something. The increased ROM in those vital areas allows the tissue to better absorb and transfer the forces encountered in sports and athletics, thus protecting the tissues and preventing injuries.

When the force of momentum is transmitted through the body, it must be properly distributed through all the tissues. The body both resists and transmits forces at the same time. The body needs sufficient reserve flexibility and range of motion to successfully handle both predictable and unpredictable forces or it is at risk for serious injury. For example, if you reach a little farther than usual to make

> Thanks to my stretching program, I always feel loose enough to go at 100 percent on the field. If I go down, I can get right back up—my flexibility makes it happen.
>
> *Donovan McNabb,*
> *Four-Time NFL Pro Bowler*
> *and client since 2000*

a tennis shot and attempt to hit it with all your power, you are putting yourself at risk for pulling a muscle or tearing some tissue if your body cannot absorb the demand of the movement. A list of potential injuries that can be avoided if the athlete has sufficient flexibility would be a very long one. A list of injuries that could be avoided by having a sufficient *reserve* of flexibility would be even longer. The bottom line is that lack of flexibility anywhere in the body eventually renders you more susceptible to injury.

If you observe the difference in the quality of movement of two athletes participating in the same sport—one who has that 20 percent reserve flexibility and one who has limited flexibility—you can clearly see how flexibility can improve athletic performance. Simply put, sport is movement, and quality of movement is either enhanced by flexibility or constrained by the lack of it.

Another advantage of having a flexibility reserve is that it protects you when you are training or competing in cold weather, when it's difficult for

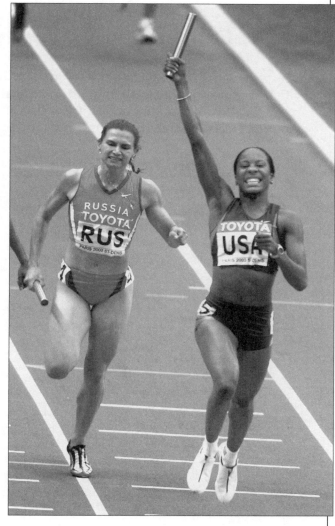

Olympic gold medalist Sanya Richards, right, credits her daily Stretch to Win routines with allowing her to compete without pain and helping her to stay injury free.

muscles and tissues to stay warm and pliable. Chances for injury are increased in those situations, but if you have reserve flexibility you can tap into it to keep your tissues ready for optimal performance.

Of all of the reasons flexibility is important in life, in sports it always comes down to just two critical ones: injury prevention and improved athletic performance. If you don't have enough flexibility in the hips and pelvis, you risk having low back problems, which is one of the most common complaints we hear from athletes when they first come to us. Once the hips and pelvis become more flexible, the low back issues often go away.

Determining Your Sport's Dominant Movement Patterns

As we discuss in chapter 6, the foundation of any matrix of stretching is the four core stretches. Because they are instrumental for movement and needed in almost all sports, athletes benefit from starting with these. Later, you can add new stretches as your analysis of your sport and circumstances dictates.

Table 7.1   Dominant Movement Patterns in Sports

	Baseball	Basketball	Cricket	Cycling	Diving	Field hockey	Figure skating	Football (American)	Golf	Gymnastics	Handball	Hockey	Jai alai	Kayaking	Lacrosse	Martial arts
Short-distance sprinting	x	x		x		x		x				x			x	
Long-distance running				x		x										
Cutting while running		x						x				x			x	
Darting while running								x			x					
Jumping		x			x		x	x		x						
Kicking								x								x
Throwing	x	x						x								
Swinging and hitting	x		x			x			x		x	x				x
Swinging, catching, and throwing	x												x		x	
Collision		x						x				x				
Specialized movements					x		x		x	x				x		

To help you build your sport-specific stretching matrix, table 7.1 lists the common movement patterns used in different sports. Finding the movements you use will help you select which stretches will be the best to prepare you for your sport. If your sport is not listed in table 7.1, determining which of the movements are used in your sport will guide you toward the most effective stretches.

The matrix is organized so that you do the four core stretches first, then add two or three or more stretches that are specific to the dominant movements in your sport and the muscle groups that you want to loosen based on the findings

	Polo	Racquetball	Rowing	Rugby	Skiing, cross-country	Skiing, downhill	Soccer	Softball	Speed skating	Squash	Swimming	Tennis	Track and field—jumping events	Track and field—long-distance events	Track and field—sprints	Track and field—throwing events	Volleyball	Weightlifting	Wrestling
				X	X	X	X	X	X		X	X	X		X				
				X					X		X			X					
				X		X	X					X							
	X			X						X									
				X										X			X		
				X			X												
				X				X									X		
	X	X						X		X		X					X		
								X											
			X																
			X		X	X			X		X							X	X

from your PFA. Frequently the dominant movement patterns in your sport will correlate with the tight muscles you found in doing your PFA.

American football is one sport that has many of the dominant movement patterns mentioned in table 7.1. For example, the running that football players do a great deal includes most of the different techniques found in other sports. There are short sprints at full speed as in track, and lateral running movement as in tennis and other racquet sports. There are runs of various distances and speeds that include cutting, darting, twisting, and jumping as in basketball, soccer, and lacrosse. Apart from running techniques, throwing the football uses the same basic overhead motion used in baseball, softball, volleyball, and the javelin in track and field. There is catching, as in many other ball sports. And for the kicker, the kicking action is similar to that in soccer and other sports where the foot makes contact with the ball or with another person, as in martial arts.

> Baseball is all about power from the core and hip movement. During the nine years I've been using the Stretch to Win system, I've had a substantial decrease in injuries and a major increase in my flexibility and strength.
>
> *Rich Aurilia,*
> *professional*
> *baseball player*

The collision component in football is also seen in hockey, rugby, and basketball. It requires total flexibility because of the uncertain and awkward positions a body can get hit in and go down in. Exceptional flexibility can also prevent many injuries in other sports in which athletes assume difficult or unusual positions such as gymnastics, diving, and wrestling.

Using the functional stretches is a good way to tailor the stretching matrix for your own custom fit, adding all the details you like. Think about the dominant movement patterns in your sports and activities. When you completed your personal flexibility assessment (PFA) in chapter 4, did you discover that you have special areas that need additional stretching because of injuries or the demands of your activities? If your low back is an area of concern, for instance, you can increase the number of stretches for that region. If you have to execute unusual movement patterns such as a breaststroke in swimming, a golf swing, or making a save as a hockey goalie, you need to choose stretches that address those particular needs. If you participate in a unilateral sport such as golf, this is where you would add one or more stretches for the opposite side of your body to balance the tissues in the body.

The following section offers some examples of stretches you can use to target specific muscles that are often used in sports.

In both short and long sprints along a straight path of travel, athletes seek to have as rapid a turnover in the legs as possible to gain the most yardage in the shortest time. We find that this ability improves in response to warm-up stretches that focus on the back and hips.

HAMSTRINGS AND LOWER BODY

1. Begin in a standing position. Inhale, and roll down to the floor on the exhale, keeping the knees bent.
2. Walk hands out, keeping the heels flat on the floor.
3. With hands and feet on the floor, press the body back toward the heels as you exhale.
4. Slowly walk the right hand, then the left hand, back toward the heels, keeping the knees straight. Press the body back toward the heels and repeat until hands and feet are close together.
5. To increase the stretch, press the chest and head toward the legs, keeping the knees completely straight.
6. With your weight on the balls of the feet, walk the hands back out away from the feet, keeping the knees straight.
7. Drop the hips to one side as you exhale. Bring them back to center position as you inhale, to the other side as you exhale, then back to the center again.
8. Walk the right hand and then the left hand back, and repeat, dropping the hips to each side.
9. Continue step 8 until the hands and feet are close together.

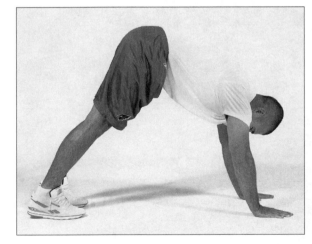 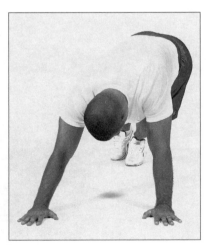

LOW BACK

1. Lie on your back. Exhale as you pull both knees into the chest. Repeat with increasing range.

2. Drop the arms out to each side and drop both legs to one side with an exhalation. Lift the legs to the center as you inhale and drop them to the other side as you exhale, repeating as necessary until you feel loose.

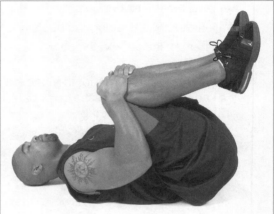

3. Roll over onto your hands and knees and slowly sit back toward the heels as you exhale, keeping your arms stretched out in front of you.

4. Tuck your chin down to your chest and continue to lower the hips down to the heels.

5. Move the hips from side to side slowly to stretch both sides of the low back.

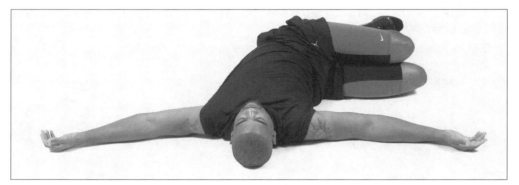

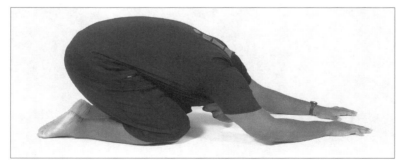

Athletes make these quick movements spontaneously, almost reflexively, based on the changing conditions at hand. In order to accomplish them with flow and coordination, the hips must have freedom of movement in as many directions as possible.

HIP RELEASE ON ALL FOURS

1. Start on your hands and knees, with the hands wider than the shoulders, fingers pointing outward, and knees together.
2. Exhale and slowly rock the hips to the right side. Inhale as you slowly return them back to center. Exhale and slowly rock the hips to the left side.
3. Alternate rocking side to side, dropping slightly farther from the center and down toward the floor, moving deeper each time.
4. To increase stretch, move the hips back toward the feet on the drop down and move them forward over the shoulder when you return to center.
5. Add moving the head to the opposite direction as you are dropping to one side to include more upper body work.
6. Continue until you feel that you have loosened up considerably and that the movement is free.

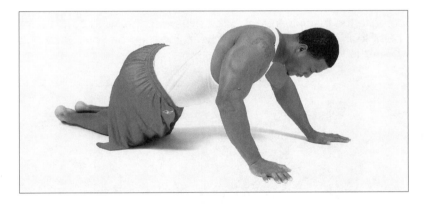

The hip flexors in the front of the body must be loose in order for the muscles engaged in backpedaling—including the glutes, the hamstrings, and the low back muscles—to fire properly. If tight hip flexors inhibit the firing of those muscles, the result will be compensations and likely eventual injury. To prevent this, the hip flexors must be released from restrictions in as many directions as possible before you do your warm-up agility drills.

SITTING HIP FLEXORS AND QUADRICEPS

1. Sit on the floor. Bring one leg to the front of the body, bending the knee and the other leg behind the body, bending the knee at a 90-degree angle. Touch the foot of the front leg to the knee of the back leg if possible.

2. Exhale and using the hands slowly move the upper body away from the front leg, moving around toward the back foot. Inhale as you release the stretch, and repeat the stretch on the exhalation.

3. To increase the stretch, on an exhalation, lift the hip slightly up off the floor, pressing the front hip higher.

4. To increase the stretch in the quadriceps, place the back forearm on the floor and bend the knee so the foot is closer to the glutes or grab the back foot with the same-side hand as the back leg.

5. To increase the fascial stretch, reach overhead the hand on the same side as the back leg, and lift the hips and keep them up as you reach outward and downward toward the floor.

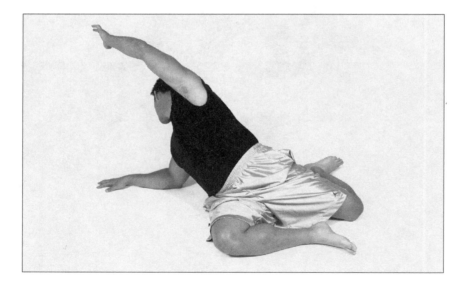

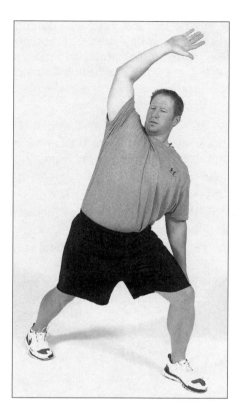

STANDING HIP FLEXORS

1. Stand in a front lunge position. Exhale as you press both hips forward, keeping the torso lifted upward.
2. Inhale as you lift overhead the arm on the same side as the back leg. Exhale as you lean to the side opposite the back leg.
3. To increase the stretch, exhale as you rotate the torso toward the ceiling and flex the hand and fingers backward.
4. Repeat the stretch until you feel loose in all areas being stretched.

PRONE HIP FLEXORS

1. Lie facedown on the floor. Press the hands and shoulders into the floor as you lift the upper body upward. Keep pressing the hips into the floor and lengthen the spine through the top of the head.
2. Lift the upper body upward as far as possible, but do not allow any pinching in the low back.
3. Press the right hip more forward and release it; continue alternating the hips back and forth several times until they feel loose.
4. To increase the stretch, lift the chin to the ceiling. To further increase the stretch and include the obliques, shift your weight more to one hand and look over the opposite shoulder. Repeat the torso rotation to the other side.

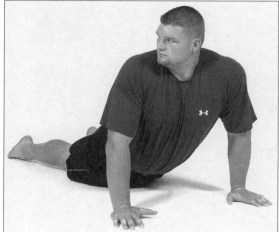

Effective jumping and leaping depend on keeping the short as well as the long muscles and their fascia free of restriction. In addition to the key stretches, adding multiple planes of movement in stretching the quadriceps, hamstrings, and calves will greatly assist you in performing these moves. It is especially important to keep the lower legs and ankles loose.

LOWER LEGS

1. Standing, bring the feet together, bend at the waist and hips with the hands on the floor and walk the hands out until the torso and the straight legs form approximately a 90-degree angle.
2. Push the hips backward and the torso down toward the floor.
3. Bending one knee slightly, press that heel into the floor releasing the other leg slightly forward with the heel coming off the floor.
4. Change to the other leg and alternate back and forth between legs until you feel loose.
5. Repeat the previous sequence but now try to straighten the back knee, continuing to alternate the movement on both sides until the lower legs feel loose.

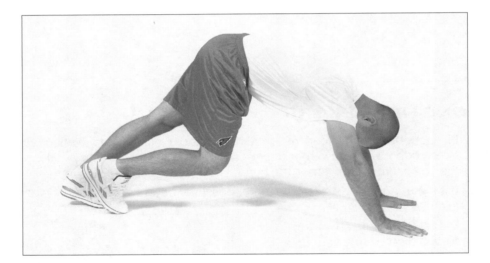

Many times the nonkicking leg experiences hamstring pulls, so incorporating both legs is important in preparing for intense kicking activities in sports. Power kicking with a dominant leg, as in American football, leads to great differences in strength and flexibility between the two sides of the body. Keeping the body balanced with an individualized flexibility warm-up will help rectify this situation. Loosening up all the hip flexors, the deep glutes, the quads, and the hamstrings is essential for effective kicking. Remember, it is the actual kick itself that must be optimized. Finish your flexibility warm-up with the kicking movement, progressively increasing the amplitude.

KICKING

1. Find a stable object such as a table or chair and hold onto it while you slowly swing your kicking leg forward and backward with a bent knee.
2. Gradually increase the height of the leg swings, then gradually increase the speed at which you are moving the leg.
3. To increase the stretch, flex the foot when the leg is in front and point the toe when the leg is in back.
4. Continue swinging the leg until the movement feels free and unrestricted.
5. Perform the same stretch on the nonkicking leg at least a few times to help balance the body.

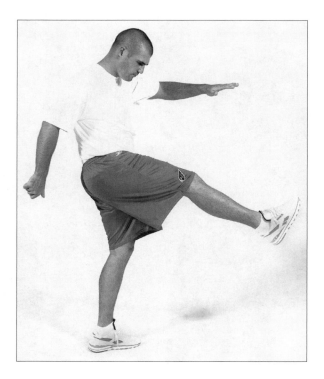

Unilateral throwing and swinging are always associated with core trunk and pelvis rotation, with the upper body rotating away from the lower body on the preparation and toward it on the release of the ball. Bilateral throwing, as done by basketball players, involves bending the spine backward with the arms flexed over and behind the head before releasing the ball with a high-velocity wavelike or whiplike motion. An essential part of throwing comes from the flexibility, strength, and stability deep within your core. Conditioning the core targets your center of gravity, located just below and deeper than your navel. Flanking your center of gravity is the iliacus and psoas group (commonly called the iliopsoas), a major part of the larger hip flexor group. They are also postural muscles, so they strongly influence how you support and stabilize your spine. Even though you are warming up to swing or throw with your arms, you must make the hips loose enough to permit the required rotation to occur.

THROWING

1. Stand with the feet about a foot apart, with the back leg slightly behind the front.
2. With a straight elbow, reach your throwing arm out to the side and open the chest as you rotate the arm and torso away from the hips.
3. Release and repeat until you feel loose.
4. Externally rotate the arm to reproduce the throwing position as you rotate the arm and torso away from the hips.
5. Repeat the movement until you feel loose in both directions.

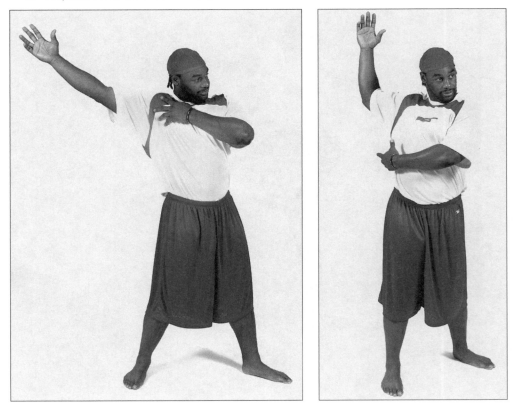

INTEGRATED HIP AND ARM STRETCH

1. Sit on the floor with one leg bent in front the body on the floor and the other leg bent behind.
2. Slide the arms out along the floor away from the legs until you feel a stretch in both the arms and hips.
3. Press the chest toward the floor as you slide the arms outward.

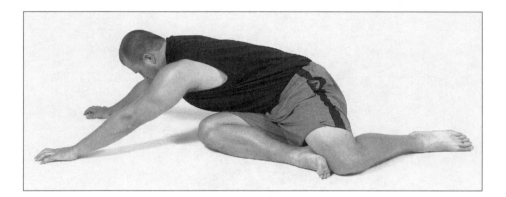

ARM AND TORSO ROTATION

1. From the starting position in the stretch above, drop down to lean on the back elbow and reach the other arm overhead.

2. Exhale and rotate the torso upward and backward.

3. Rotate the torso back down toward the floor.

4. Circle the top arm as far around as possible in both directions as you repeat the movement until it feels smooth.

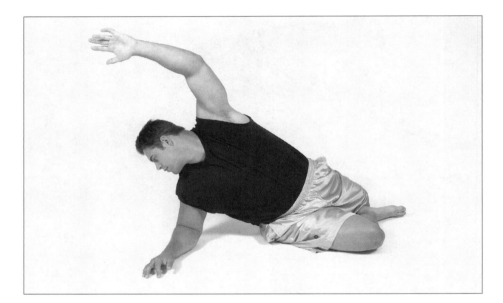

Choosing Your Tempo

The best approach to building a solid flexibility program involves three stages. First, you should develop your passive flexibility using the slower tempos (SW_{VS} and SW_S; refer back to chapter 5, pages 109 to 111) to get that 20 percent reserve flexibility. Then, move on to developing more active flexibility with the fast tempo (SW_F; see page 111), which will help you function in activities of daily living and in some slower-paced sports. When you have accomplished those goals, it's time to develop your ability to flow through your athletic movements very quickly using the very fast tempos (SW_{VF}, page 112). As we discuss in chapter 5, what is commonly referred to as ballistic stretching we call doing the stretch wave very fast—a rapid tempo with increased power and momentum behind it. This type of stretching is used to prepare for many sports, but it is best not to engage in it until you are experienced with the slower stretch waves.

While you can see some gains in flexibility in as little as a few hours using the slow or very slow stretching, many gains can be made in four to six weeks of following a regular program. Also, gains in flexibility are cumulative so as you continue your stretching program, your flexibility should get better and better, and after a few months you should see substantial gains.

Of all the kinds of stretching in this system, SW_{VF} is the most closely related to the actual athletic movements you will be performing, and it uses the most force and velocity. By the time you finish this type of stretching, you should be very warmed up and ready to start your activity. This kind of warm-up is especially important if the activity involves power moves that require great speed and force. When conducted at the right time in your flexibility training program, stretching with a quicker tempo has a strong beneficial effect on your connective tissues, giving you the extra edge you need for optimal performance.

While all athletes should warm up first with light cardiovascular work followed by stretches and exercises that are similar to the movements they use in their given sports, not all do. We have found that a specific SW_{VF} stretch routine that targets the areas of the body that will be used in the sport has often provided the missing link in our clients' training routines. For instance, one of our Olympic gold-medal winning pole-vaulters balanced out her training by practicing sprints carrying her pole on the opposite side from usual. This relieved the stress accumulating on her dominant side and ultimately helped to realign her posture. It was so effective that she made it part of her permanent warm-up stretch routine.

Sample Stretch Wave Program

Here's a good overall fast stretch wave program that athletes engaging in most sports can perform as a SW_F program before their activity or event. Perform these stretches on a field or indoors. All of these stretches can also be done at a slower tempo or a very fast tempo.

HIP CIRCLES

1. Stand with the feet hip-distance apart and the hands on the hips.
2. Push the hips out to the right side and circle them around to the back, then left, front, to the right once more, and so on. Begin with small, slow circles and gradually increase their size and speed.
3. Continue circles until the hips feel loose in every direction.
4. Reverse the direction of the circles and continue until the hips feel loose in every direction moving this way as well.

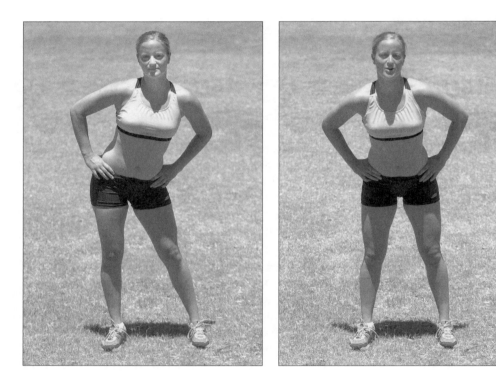

HIP SERIES—KNEELING

1. Kneel on one leg, place the hands on the front knee or on the hips, and lunge forward over the front leg, making sure the bent knee is at a 90-degree angle and does not lean past the toes.

2. Press both hips forward and keep the chest lifted. Move in and out of the stretch until the hip flexor feels loose.

3. Push the hips out to one side, moving them toward the left if your left knee is the back knee, or toward the right if the back knee is on that side. Bend the torso away from the hip being stretched.

4. Bend the head and torso forward to release the stretch and come up to the starting position. Repeat the sequence until you feel loose.

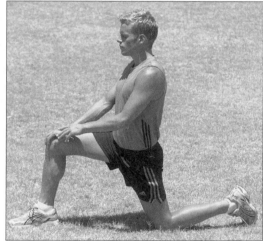

5. Now open the front leg out to the side, keeping the knee bent and the foot on the ground.

6. Lunge toward the outside of the upright leg and hip, leaning away from the kneeling leg and hip.

7. Wave in and out of the stretch, rocking from side to side until you feel more loose in the hip flexors, lateral hip, and adductors.

8. Repeat the series on the other side.

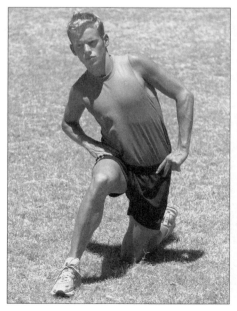

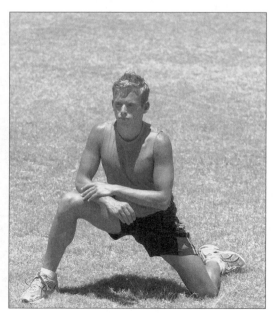

LEG SWINGS

1. Standing up, swing one leg forward and backward, keeping the knee bent. Swing the arms in opposition to the swinging leg. Begin with small and slow movements and gradually increase their size and speed; continue until the hips feel loose. Repeat on the other side.

2. Straighten the knee and flex the foot as you again swing the leg from front to back, moving the arms in opposition. Increase the size and speed of swings

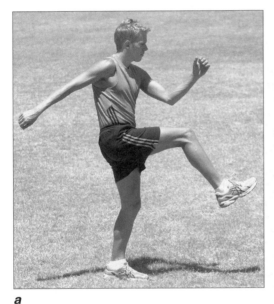

a

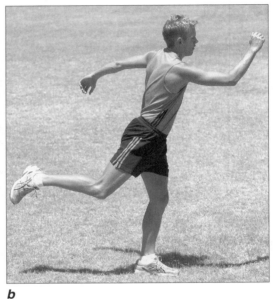

b

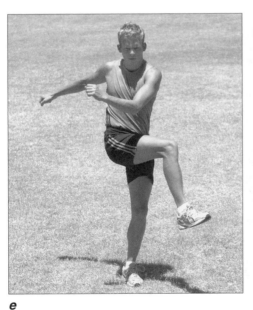

e

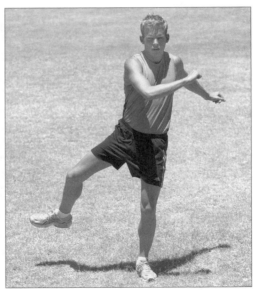

f

and continue until the leg feels loose in both directions. Repeat on the other side.

3. Now swing the leg across the body and out to the side, keeping the knee bent. Move the arms across torso in opposition to the leg movement. Once again, begin with small and slow movements and increase the size and speed of the swings until you feel loose in both directions. Repeat on the other side.

4. Repeat the previous swing, but this time with the swinging leg straight and the foot flexed, until you feel loose in both directions. Repeat on the other side.

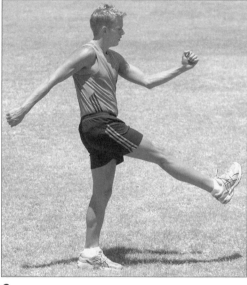

c

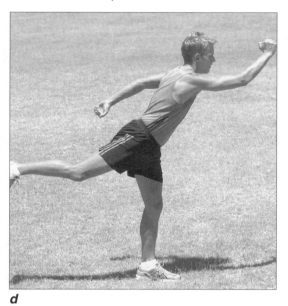

d

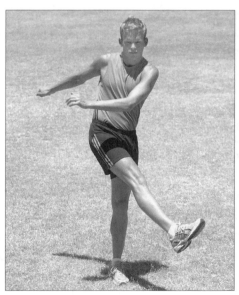

g

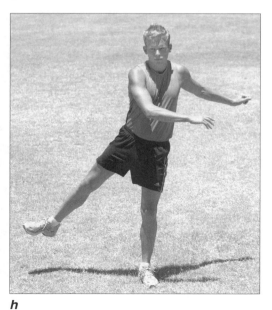

h

GLUTES—STANDING

1. From a standing position, cross one ankle over the other leg above the knee and bend the standing knee.
2. Bend at the hips and touch the ground with the fingertips.
3. Increase the bend of the standing knee to deepen the stretch. Move in and out of this position until glutes feel loose.
4. Repeat on the other side.

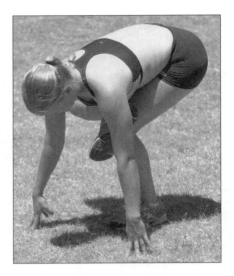

ABDOMINALS

1. Lie facedown with the top of the feet resting on the ground. Bend the arms and place the hands on the floor beneath the shoulders, palms down, with fingers pointing away from the body.
2. Press the hands and shoulders into the ground as you lift the upper body upward. Keep pressing the hips into the ground and lengthen the spine through the top of the head, pulling the abdomen in slightly.
3. Lift the upper body as far as possible, but do not allow any pinching in the low back. To increase the stretch, lift the chin.
4. To further increase the stretch and include the obliques, shift your weight more to one hand and look over the opposite shoulder.
5. Repeat the torso rotation to the other side.

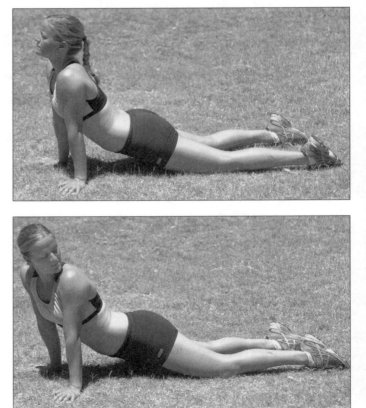

QUADRATUS LUMBORUM AND ILIOTIBIAL BAND

1. Lie on the ground on your side. Bend the top leg and cross it over the bottom leg such that the foot of the top leg is on the ground.
2. Placing the hands on the ground and straightening the arms for support, raise your torso off the ground.
3. Slide the bottom leg away from the top leg, keeping the top leg in place.
4. Keeping the torso upright and the bottom hip on the ground, wave the hips by slightly rolling the pelvis forward and backward. To increase the stretch, lift the torso up more and slide the bottom leg farther from the torso.
5. Repeat on the other side.

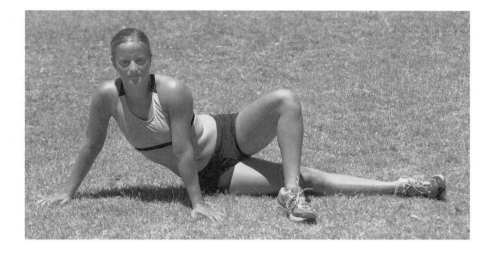

LOW BACK

1. Lie on your back. Pull both knees into the chest and hug them with both arms.
2. Tuck the chin toward the chest and lift the hips off the ground.
3. Rock back and forth, very slowly at first and then increasing the speed and size of the movement.
4. Keeping the knees together, drop the legs over to one side, then separate them 8 to 12 inches (20 to 30 centimeters), with one knee placed higher than the other.

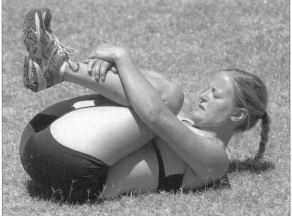

5. Squeeze the knees together again, tighten the abdominals, and pull the legs back up into the original position.
6. Drop the legs down on the other side and repeat steps 4 and 5 on that side. Continue alternating between sides until the low back feels loose.

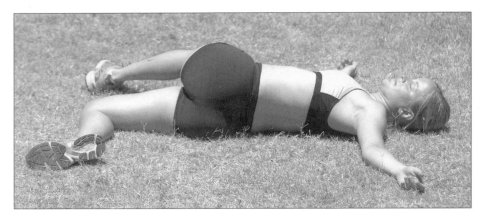

GLUTES—LYING

1. Lie on your back—if possible, at a pole or a wall. If a pole or wall is available, place one foot on it off the ground; if not available, plant one foot on the ground with the knee bent at 90 degrees.
2. Bend the other knee and place that ankle above the knee of the planted leg. Support the bent knee and the ankle with the hands.
3. Push the knee away from the body to stretch the hip flexors and the deep rotators of the leg. Release, then repeat as needed.
4. Next, pull the top leg toward the chest with both hands, keeping it bent at a 90-degree angle until you feel the stretch. To increase stretch, you can reach under the bottom leg and pull both legs toward the chest.
5. Bring the knee of the top leg to the center line of the body and pull it down into the chest. Simultaneously, grab the ankle and bring it down toward the floor with the opposite hand.
6. Roll the body to the side of the bottom leg to increase the stretch.
7. Explore the different angles and fibers by rocking the body slightly from side to side.
8. To increase the stretch, move the knee to the opposite shoulder and pull the ankle to the floor
9. Repeat the entire sequence on the other side.

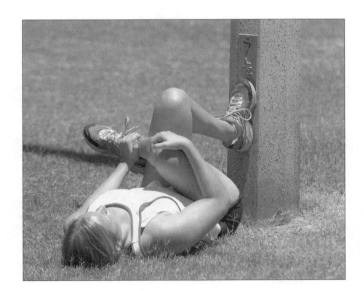

HAMSTRINGS

1. Stand with the feet 2 to 4 feet apart (61 to 122 cm) and bend both knees.
2. Bend at the hips and grab the ankles.
3. Gently try to straighten the legs.
4. Release stretch and bend the knees again. Repeat until the hamstrings and hips feel loose.
5. Shift weight over to the right side and try to straighten the legs, releasing when the stretch sensation prevents any more movement. Then do the same on the left side. Keep moving from side to side, repeating until the hamstrings feel loose.

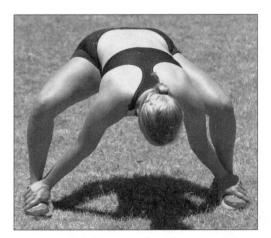

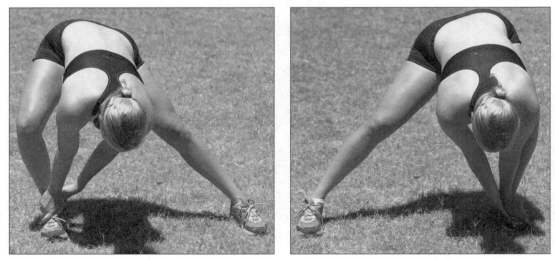

LOWER LEGS

1. Stand with feet a comfortable distance apart, then bend at the waist and touch the ground with the hands.
2. Bring the feet together and walk the hands out on the ground until the torso and the straight legs form approximately a 90-degree angle.
3. Push the hips back and the torso down toward the ground.
4. Bending one knee slightly, press that heel into the ground, releasing the other leg slightly forward with the heel coming off the ground.
5. Change to the other leg and alternate back and forth between legs until you feel loose.
6. Repeat the previous sequence but now try to straighten the back knee, continuing the movement on both sides until the lower legs feel loose.

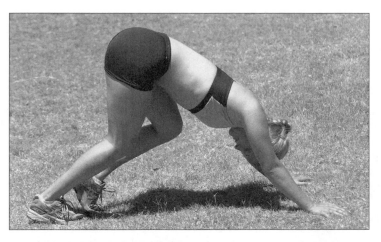

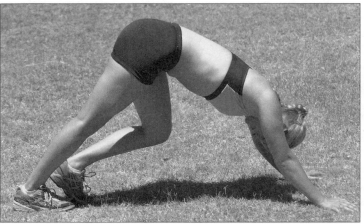

LATERAL LINE

1. Standing with the feet hip-width apart, inhale and raise one arm over the head.

2. Exhale and bend as far as possible to the side opposite the raised arm. Stretch through the fingertips.

3. Explore different angles by gently rotating the torso down toward the ground and then upward, repeating until you feel it loosening up. To increase the stretch, turn the top arm so the palm is facing upward and grab the top hand with the hand of the bottom arm.

4. Now roll from the side stretch position down to the center of the body and through to the other side.

5. Stretch from side to side, moving through the center of the body until both sides feel loose.

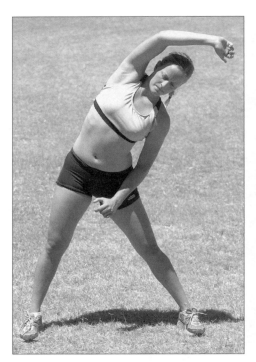 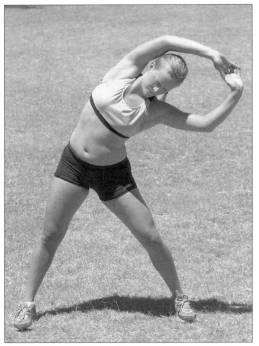

ARM SWINGS

1. Stand with the feet hip-distance apart.
2. Swing the arms back and forth, moving one to the front while the other goes back. Slowly increase the size and speed of the movement and continue until the arms and shoulders feel loose.
3. Swing the arms across the chest and over the head, still alternating them, and continue each movement until the arms and shoulders feel loose.

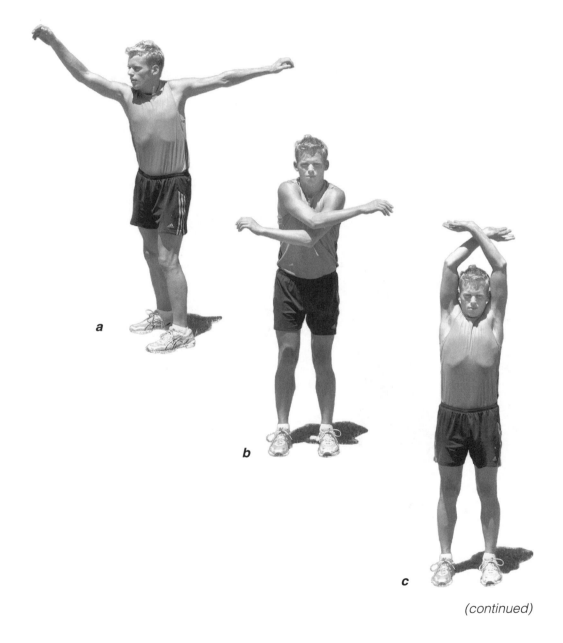

a

b

c

(continued)

(continued)

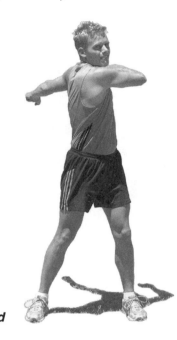

4. With knees slightly bent, swing the arms across the body with the torso rotating from side to side. Bring the front arm across the body as far as possible and the back arm as far back as possible while rotating the torso as far as possible.

5. Slowly increasing the size and speed of the movement, continue until the arms, shoulders, and torso feel loose.

6. Bend at the waist and drop the torso toward the floor; continue the swinging movement until it feels loose.

7. Alternate keeping the head centered for several swings and turning it to initiate the rotation of the torso and arms.

d

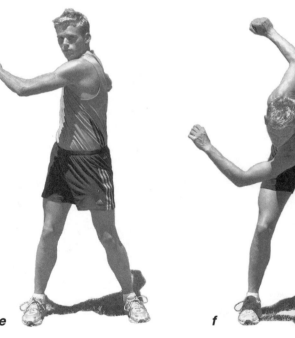

e

f

ARM SERIES

This series targets the shoulders, the biceps, and the wrist flexors and extensors.

1. Stand with the feet hip-width apart. Take the arms out to the sides and bend the elbows at a 90-degree angle, with the fingers pointing upward.

2. Externally rotate the shoulders back as far as possible, then internally rotate them as far down as possible, always keeping the 90-degree elbow angle. Continue alternating external and internal rotation until the shoulders feel loose.

3. Take the arms straight out to sides and alternate turning the palms upward and downward, rotating the shoulders as far as possible with each movement. You can also alternate the arms in opposite directions.

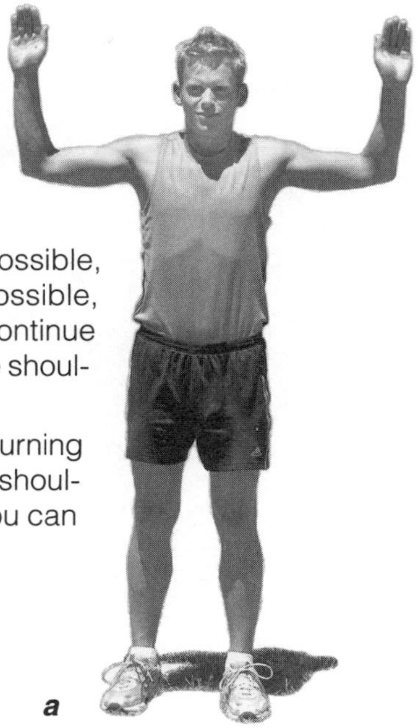

a

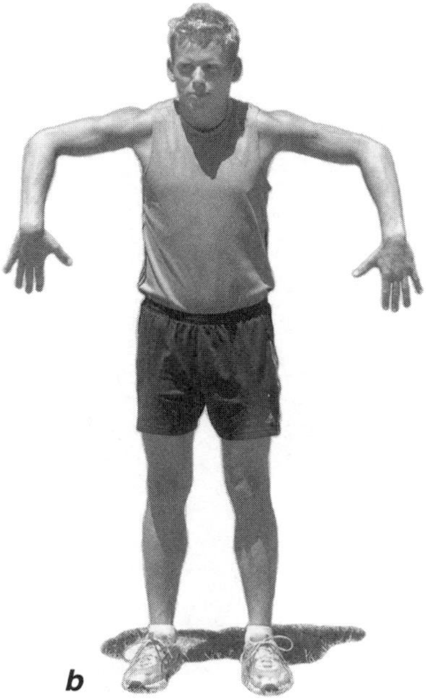

b

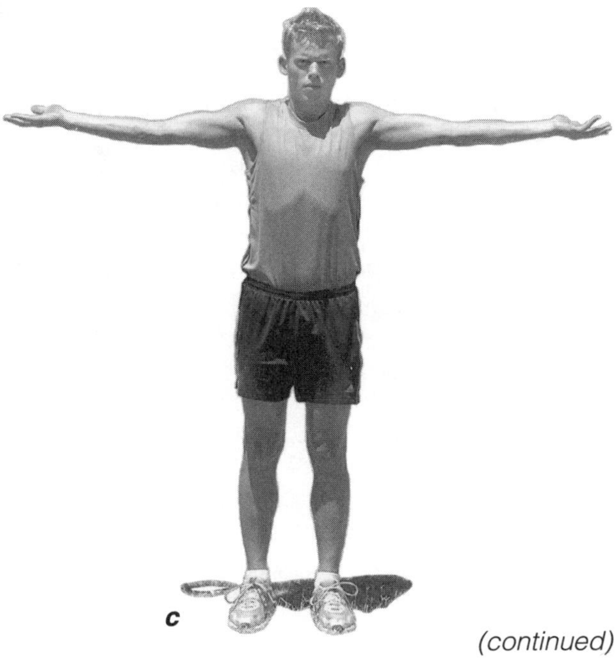

c

(continued)

(continued)

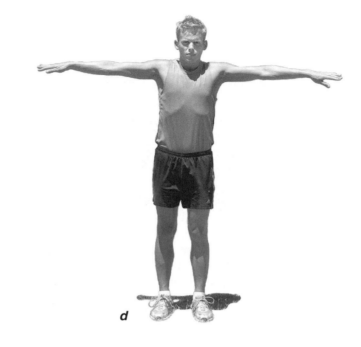

d

5. Stand up straight and exhale as you gently pull the arm across the back as far as possible. To increase the stretch, push the hand you are stretching away from the low back or bend the head into lateral flexion away from the shoulder of the arm being pulled.

6. Move in and out of the stretch until you feel loose.

7. Relax the arm down into its socket again, and draw it across the chest with the other hand, keeping the elbow straight. Use the assisting arm to bring the arm being stretched toward the body.

e

f

8. Bring the stretched arm as far across the chest as far as possible, keeping the elbow as straight as possible. To increase the stretch, change the position of the assisting arm to hold above the wrist and straighten the arm as you continue to bring it across and into the chest. Exhale as you gently pull the arm across the chest, making sure the shoulder stays in the socket.

9. Move in and out of the stretch until you feel loose.

10. Now gently traction the wrist out by grasping the hand with other hand. Place your hands palm to palm with the hand of the wrist being stretched resting on the bottom, its fingers pointing in the same direction (downward) as the assisting hand's. Relax the elbow and shoulder as you flex the fingertips and thumb toward the body. To increase the stretch, slide the top hand down so that its fingertips meet those of the assisting hand and straighten the elbow.

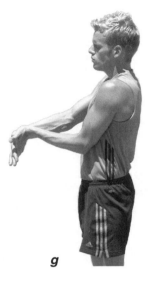

g

11. Explore different angles by moving the hand toward the thumb and then toward the pinkie.

12. Now lift one arm behind you and turn the hand with the back of the wrist facing downward. Internally rotate the arm slightly from the shoulder all the way down to the thumb.

13. Bend the wrist toward the palm, reaching the fingers upward. To increase the stretch, turn the body and head away from the arm and exhale into the stretch.

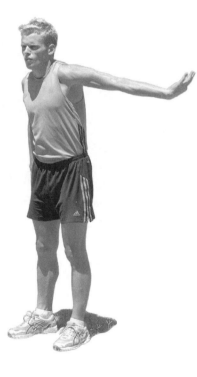

h

chapter 8

Assisted Stretching Routines

The main focus of the stretches and programs presented in this book is self-stretching, but there are also many stretches you can do with the assistance of a trained professional. Assisted stretching allows you to take advantage of the power of another person in a relaxed environment to increase your range of motion without pain. When athletes at our clinic have stretched this way they've found it enormously effective and motivating, and you can experience the same benefits. While all 10 of the Stretch to Win principles apply to assisted stretching as well, a few of them are especially relevant—principles 7 ("Target the entire joint"; see page 11), 8 ("Use traction"; see page 12), and 9 ("Facilitate body reflexes"—proprioceptive neuromuscular facilitation; see page 14). While none of the assisted stretches presented in this chapter are high-risk, it is always best to have a stretching partner who has some background in anatomy and physiology, ideally a trainer, physical therapist, or massage therapist. Without the proper background, sometimes coaches or other athletes can stretch too aggressively.

As you'll recall from chapter 1, the joint capsule is a secure connective-tissue bag that surrounds and holds our bones together where they meet at the joints. It can contribute to up to 50 percent of your lack of ROM at the joint. When the capsule gets tight, it often adheres, or gets "glued down," to the bone. Until you address this situation, you will be neglecting a major cause of inflexibility. It stands to reason, then, that including the joint capsule in stretching is a must to maximize your functional ROM. In this chapter we provide guidelines for when stretching the joint capsule is indicated or contraindicated based on your individual condition, and we tell you how to implement it within a partner-assisted stretching program.

Traction is an important piece of the puzzle in getting the joint capsule to stretch. As we state in chapter 1, after getting the joint capsule optimally mobile, the next focus is to traction and stretch the muscles that cross only one joint. Because these muscles are shorter and closer to the joint than the muscles that cross two joints, it is necessary to release them first; this paves the way for the longer muscles to release more quickly and efficiently. When we get to stretching the two-joint muscles, we add traction proximally and distally to get a complete myofascial stretch from the origin of the muscle to its insertion. In fact, traction goes beyond local muscular attachments and on to related proximal and distal fascial lines, amplifying the effect of stretching.

The great significance of traction in assisted stretching is that it increases the level of relaxation through the joint receptors and significantly reduces pain by aiding the release of endorphins, nature's own pain reliever. When the body's natural pain relievers and muscle relaxants are stimulated from the stretching, they are released into the bloodstream and travel throughout the body, making you more relaxed and facilitating even better results. Traction makes all the difference for maximal lengthening of the connective tissue.

Traction also eliminates the "jamming" sensation in joints that is so common when an athlete is being stretched by another person. You can observe a glaring example of this on an athletic field when a well-meaning trainer or therapist is unknowingly pushing an athlete's femoral head deeper into the hip joint during a straight-leg hamstring stretch with the athlete lying on his or her back. It is not uncommon to actually see the athlete wincing in pain and squirming to get away as the soft tissue structures of the hip are compressed and pinched. Well-placed traction avoids this and makes stretching much more comfortable.

You can use accessories if self-stretching using proprioceptive neuromuscular facilitation (PNF), but assisted PNF is especially effective with the help of a trainer, therapist, or a trusted partner. Our adapted version, called undulating PNF, is different from the traditional method for several reasons. It is important to have a solid understanding of our adapted technique in order to perform it correctly and maximize results with assisted stretching. To clarify, we use what is commonly known as the contract-relax method, but we also bring in our principles 7 and 8. The outside force of a partner allows for greater traction of the joint capsule, which is a crucial component for eliminating one of the largest restrictive factors to optimal flexibility. We believe in using slight traction before progressing with any assisted stretching.

Another difference in our undulating PNF technique is the way we use breathing to time the stretch. As with our other types of stretching, instead of using a set amount of time, we use the inhalation of the person being stretched, which lasts about three to four seconds. We also believe it is better to use a moderate isometric contraction of between 25 and 50 percent of strength, instead of a maximal contraction; that is, before the stretch, the athlete contracts the muscles to be stretched to 25 to 50 percent of full strength. It is also important to slowly increase and decrease the contraction in a smooth and controlled manner. After the contraction, the partner gently tractions the joint out of the socket and then increases the stretch on the exhalation. We highly recommend using this undulating PNF style for making major flexibility gains, instead of the typical jerky approach—it's much easier on the partner and more enjoyable for the person being stretched. It is important to always move in a smooth and gentle manner and have a coordinated rhythm together. This will be the most effective type of stretching in any flexibility training session. CRAC, an acronym for contract (isometric contraction of the antagonist) and relax, followed by an agonist contraction, is another highly effective technique, which we use in special sequences beyond the scope of this book.

The last aspect of our assisted stretching technique that makes it unique is our use of restraining straps. When we were developing this method, the necessity of creating some kind of leverage was obvious, especially given the size and strength of the athletes with whom we were working. Our restraining straps have progressed from uncomfortable seat belt-type material to cushioned belts that can slide easily under our specialized tables.

Figure 8.1a shows a good example of the awkwardness and lack of control of an assisted stretch done without the restraining straps, while figure 8.1b shows the level of control we can attain by using the restraining straps. Our professional NFL clients are the models for the photos in this chapter, as they are in chapter 7 and some of the stretches in chapter 6. You may notice a slight difference between the size of the athlete and the size of one of the flexibility specialists!

All these stretches can use the slow, fast, or undulating PNF tempos, depending on the circumstance. If it is pre-event, or "go time," as we call it, then a fast undulating tempo is needed. To get the athlete ready for action and full-speed movement it is necessary to pick up the pace a bit. However, we do not use a very fast tempo with assisted stretching; it is reserved for self-stretching immediately before activity or an event. If it is postevent or after activity, it's time for recovery, which dictates a slow or very slow undulating tempo to calm down the body and mind and restore the flexibility lost to intense athletic participation.

If an athlete feels tighter on one side of the body, you can help balance out his or her flexibility by using a two-to-one ratio—stretch the tighter side first, then the other side, then the tighter side again. The best guide is to feel the tissue and listen to your instincts. It is always better to stretch less and allow the athlete's body to relax before you proceed. Assisted stretching is a partnership between the assister and the athlete.

It is just amazing how such a little lady can stretch someone as big as I am and never even break a sweat—and it's so smooth, like she is dancing with me.

Fred Wakefield, NFL player, 315-pound (154 kg), 6-foot-7-inch (203 cm) offensive tackle

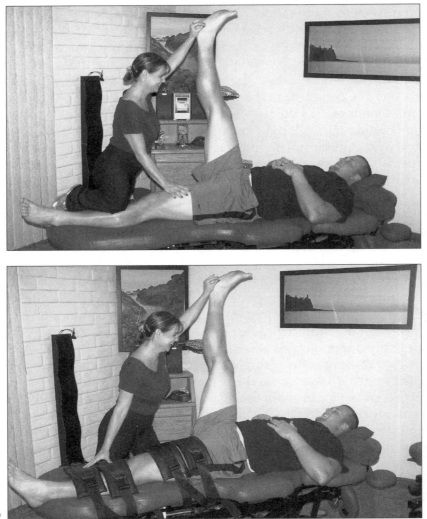

Figure 8.1 Without table straps *(a)*, the practitioner must manually stabilize the client; this is awkward, and it puts the practitioner at risk for cumulative stress and strain. The Stretch to Win table straps *(b)* completely stabilize the part of the body not being stretched, allowing the practitioner to have superior leverage and to focus more fully on the part of the body being stretched.

Lower Body Assisted Stretches—Floor

The stretches shown in this section apply to most sports. As with all stretching programs, it's important when developing an assisted stretching program to keep in mind the concept of most athletic movement being initiated from the hips. These stretches are designed in a specific routine and can be done together—one right after the other—or separately. After you have completed the routine on one leg, repeat the sequence on the other leg.

LOW BACK

1. The athlete lies on the back. The assister bends the athlete's top leg and crosses it over the bottom leg.
2. The assister slides one foot into the crook of the athlete's back knee and gently moves the athlete's knee up toward the athlete's shoulder; traction is out and up. The assister's leg braces the athlete's other leg. The athlete tries to keep the opposite shoulder down.
3. For PNF, the athlete presses into the assister's front leg by contracting the hamstrings.
4. The assister gently tractions the athlete's top leg out and moves it away from the bottom leg on the exhalation to increase the stretch.
5. Repeat two more times and explore different angles of the stretch.

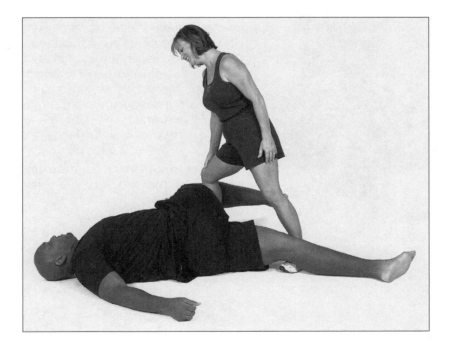

GLUTEUS MAXIMUS AND DEEP ROTATORS

1. From the low back stretch, the athlete rolls flat onto the back, bringing the leg to a 90-degree angle across the body.

2. The assister holds the athlete with one hand on the athlete's heel and the other in front of the bent knee to externally rotate the athlete's femur and to bring the foot toward the opposite shoulder. The athlete's foot rests on the assister's shoulder.

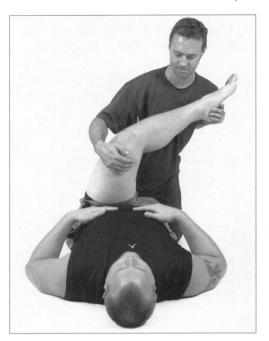

3. For PNF, the assister moves his or her hand to the back side of the athlete's knee, and the athlete gently pushes into the assister's hand.

4. As the athlete exhales, the assister tractions the hip gently up and out of the athlete's socket and slowly increases the stretch by bringing the athlete's femur toward the chest. The closer the leg is to the chest, the deeper the stretch in the gluteus maximus. The more the leg externally rotates, the deeper the stretch in the rotators.

5. Repeat two or more times and explore different angles of the stretch.

GLUTEUS MEDIUS

1. The assister brings the athlete's knee to the center of the chest and moves the foot down toward the opposite hip.
2. For PNF, the athlete presses the knee into the assister's hand.
3. As the athlete exhales, the assister tractions the athlete's hip gently upward and out of the socket before increasing the hip flexion and adduction. If there is pinching in the front of the hip, the assister applies more focus on the foot.
4. Repeat two or more times and explore different angles of the stretch.

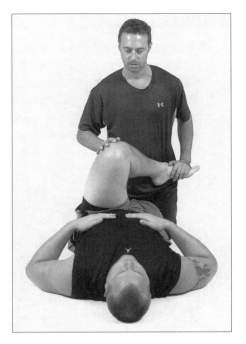

LATERAL HAMSTRINGS

1. The assister extends the athlete's leg out and crosses it over the body. The athlete should keep the knee bent if necessary, and the assister can traction the leg up and out of the hip socket.
2. For PNF, the athlete pushes with the entire leg against the assister's leg.
3. As the athlete exhales, the assister gently tractions the athlete's leg up and out of the socket using a lunging

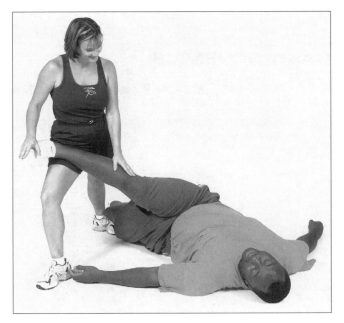

movement. The assister can increase the stretch by moving the athlete's leg deeper in lateral flexion toward the opposite shoulder and down to the floor.
4. Repeat two or more times and explore different angles of the stretch.

SOLEUS

1. The assister bends the athlete's knee and dorsiflexes the foot. The assister places a forearm under the athlete's foot and places a hand under the athlete's heel, tractioning it out.
2. For PNF, the athlete presses the ball of the foot into the arm.
3. To continue the PNF, the assister gently tractions the athlete's heel out and stretches the soleus by using the forearm to move the athlete's toes toward the shin.

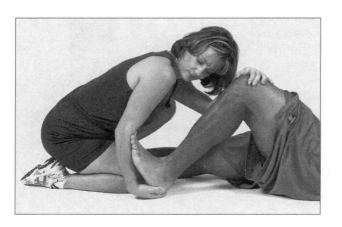

4. To increase the stretch, the assister adds downward pressure on the bottom of the athlete's femur toward the shin and continues using the forearm to move the athlete's toes toward the shin.
5. Repeat two or more times and explore different angles of the stretch by positioning the foot slightly inward or outward.

GASTROCNEMIUS

1. The assister straightens the athlete's knee outward and places a hand behind the athlete's knee.
2. The assister gently tractions the entire leg, grasping (not pinching) the athlete's heel with the other hand.

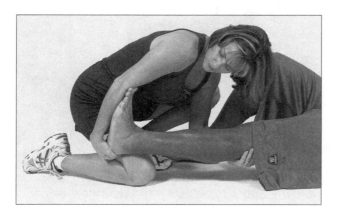

3. For PNF, the athlete gently presses the ball of his or her foot into the assister's arm.
4. The assister gently tractions the heel out and uses the forearm to stretch the gastrocnemius by moving the toes toward the shin, increasing the traction as the stretch increases.
5. Repeat two or more times and explore different angles.

HIP FLEXORS

1. The athlete gets into a deep lunge using a ball against a wall, if possible, to support the torso.
2. The assister places one hand above the knee of the athlete's back leg and the other hand on the top of the foot of the athlete's back leg to traction the leg to assure the leg is in extension to begin.
3. For PNF, the athlete pushes straight back into the assister's top hand (which is under the athlete's glute) by contracting the glutes. On the stretch, as the athlete exhales, the assister presses downward with the top hand into the back of the athlete's thigh, toward the ball, if one is being used, or the floor. The assister tractions with the hand on top of the athlete's foot to deepen the stretch as the athlete presses the hips toward the ball or the floor.
4. Repeat two or more times and explore different angles of the stretch.
5. To target the lateral aspect of hip flexors, the assister moves the top hand placement medially and changes angle of the athlete's lower leg medially. The athlete pushes back medially into the assister's top hand. For the stretch, the assister presses into the medial aspect of the athlete's ischial tuberosity and tractions the lower leg medially as the athlete presses the hips into the ball or toward the floor.
7. To target the medial aspect of the hip flexors, the assister moves the top hand placement laterally and changes the angle of the athlete's lower leg laterally. For PNF, the athlete pushes back laterally against the top hand. For the stretch, the assister presses into medial aspect of the athlete's ischial tuberosity and tractions the lower leg laterally as the athlete presses the hips toward the ball or floor.
8. Repeat two or more times and explore different angles of the stretch.

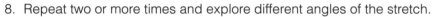

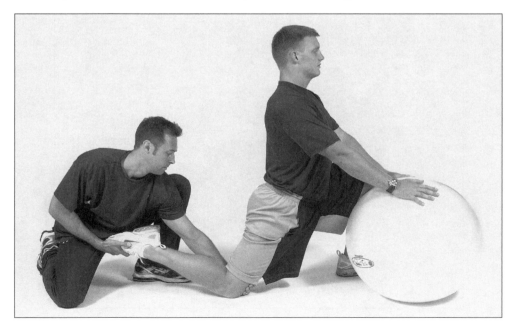

LATERAL HIP AND IT BAND

1. With the athlete lying on his or her back, the assister takes the athlete's legs over to one side so that the lower leg being stretched is just slightly off the ground and under the top leg.

2. The assister places the outside of the leg being stretched on the inside of the assister's leg above the athlete's ankle.

3. The assister lifts the athlete's top leg upward and moves it slightly across the body.

4. The athlete reaches upward with the same arm and hand as the leg being stretched.

5. For PNF, the athlete pushes against the assister's leg.

6. For the stretch, the assister increases the traction and the lateral flexion of the bottom leg.

7. Repeat two or more times and explore different angles of the stretch.

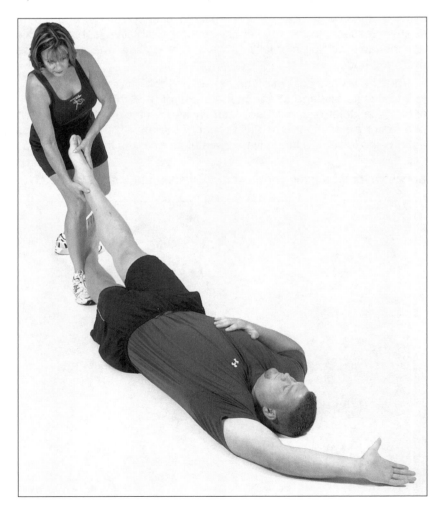

Upper Body Assisted Stretches— Sitting and Standing

Assisted stretching for the upper body can be very effective, but it must be done with more caution. The neck, especially, is a delicate structure and stretching it must be approached in a slow and gentle manner. The shoulder was designed with mobility first and stability second, so it is important not to stretch it too aggressively.

We have found that instead of completing this entire routine on one side and then repeating it on the other, it flows better if you do each stretch on both sides of the body before moving on to the next one in the routine. These stretches can all be done separately, but when combined, they hit most of the areas that need to be targeted in the upper body.

NECK

1. The athlete sits on a chair. The assister stands behind the athlete and moves the athlete's head toward one shoulder by placing one hand on the opposite shoulder and the other hand on the side of the athlete's head.

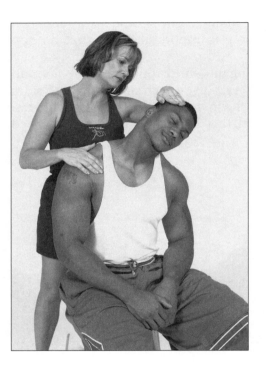

2. The assister pushes down on the athlete's opposite shoulder, moving the head the other way. The athlete's head should not tilt backward.

3. For PNF, the athlete tries to gently push the head into the assister's hand or to shrug the shoulder into the assister's other hand.

4. For the stretch, as the athlete exhales, the assister presses down firmly on the athlete's shoulder while gently increasing the athlete's lateral neck flexion.

5. The assister releases the shoulder and moves the athlete's head slowly down through neutral to the chest before starting on the other side.

6. Repeat the PNF series two or more times and explore different angles of the stretch.

ANTERIOR SHOULDER

1. The athlete sits on a bench and the assister stands behind the athlete. The assister wraps his or her arms around and above the athlete's elbows and gently squeezes them together.

2. For PNF, the athlete attempts to pull the elbows apart.

3. On the exhalation, the athlete squeezes the elbows closer together while lifting the chest up for the stretch.

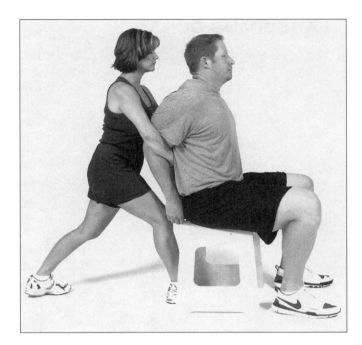

4. Repeat two or more times and explore different angles of the stretch.

CHEST

1. The athlete sits in a chair with the feet on floor and interlaces the fingers behind the head. The assister stands behind the athlete and places his or her hands around and on the outside of the athlete's elbows. The athlete can arch back a bit.

2. For PNF, the athlete tries to bring the elbows together toward the face.

3. As the athlete exhales, the assister gently tractions the athlete's elbows upward and outward away from the chest, increasing the stretch by opening the chest and arching the back slightly.

4. The assister can change the angle to stretch different pectoralis fibers by gently lifting the athlete's elbows higher.

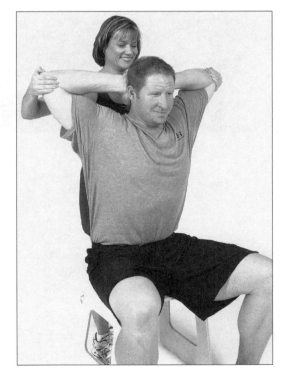

5. Repeat two or more times and explore different angles of the stretch.

LATISSIMUS DORSI

1. The athlete sits on a table with the knees bent and the feet on the floor. The assister tractions the athlete's arm upward and then bends it at the elbow.

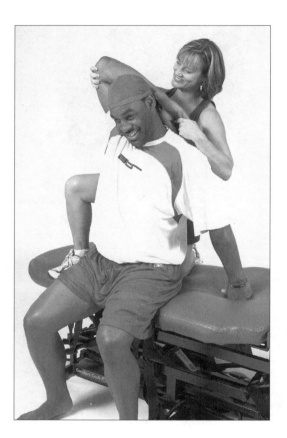

2. The assister stands or kneels behind the athlete and places one hand above the athlete's elbow and grasps the athlete's fingertips with the other hand.

3. For PNF, the athlete pushes the elbow into the assister's hand and bends the torso over to the side and down toward the floor. Another PNF option is for the athlete to attempt to bring the elbow down to the opposite knee.

4. For the stretch, as the athlete exhales, the assister tractions the bent arm upward and increases the athlete's side bend of the torso in the opposite direction. To increase the stretch, the assister can move one hand to the athlete's rib cage and keep the other hand above the athlete's elbow to rotate the chest up to the ceiling, allowing for a slight arch in the back.

5. Repeat the PNF series two or more times and explore different angles of the stretch. Repeat on the other side.

BICEPS

1. The athlete sits on a bench with the knees bent and the feet on the floor. The assister stands behind the athlete and gently tractions both arms behind the athlete with the forearms supinated. The assister holds onto the athlete's hands but leaves the thumbs free.
2. For PNF, the athlete attempts a bicep curl with both arms.
3. For the stretch, the assister lengthens the athlete's arms back outward and internally rotates (pronates) the forearms as far as comfortably possible.
4. Repeat the PNF series two or more times and explore different angles of the stretch.

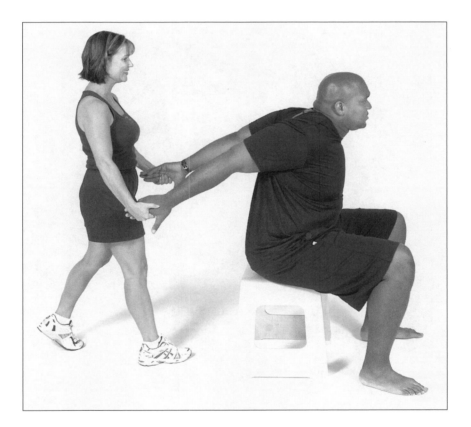

MID UPPER BACK—RHOMBOIDS

1. From a standing position, the athlete bends at the hips and reaches through with the outside arm to grasp the assister's wrist and places the other hand on the assister's shoulder. The assister places one hand on the athlete's latissimus dorsi and the other hand on the athlete's wrist.

2. On the exhalation, the athlete pulls his or her arm and shoulder back across the body and rotates away.

3. For the stretch, the assister pushes the athlete's lat upward while pulling the athlete's arm across the body, rotating the athlete's body toward the assister.

4. Repeat two or more times, exploring different angles of the stretch. Repeat with the other arm.

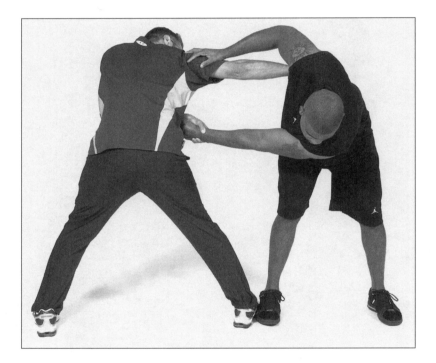

Lower Body Assisted Stretches—
Treatment Table

The specialized treatment tables we use in our clinic are designed specifically for bodywork and stretching. They have adjustable strapping belts attached to a bar under the pads that can slide to fit the size of the person being stretched. When we teach our technique at our institute we provide restraining straps that can be used on any massage or training table.

This quick routine gets the hips open and mobile in a short time and is effective for restoration or right before an activity, depending on the tempo you use. Perform all the stretches on one leg and then do the routine once more on the other leg.

LOW BACK

1. The athlete lies on his or her back with one leg restrained. The assister stands beside the table on the restrained leg side

2. The assister brings the athlete's nonrestrained leg across the athlete's body and allows the hips to rotate.

3. The assister wraps the athlete's leg across the front of the assister's body and rests it in the crease of the assister's hips, keeping the athlete's knee slightly bent.

4. The assister cradles the athlete's leg with one arm, placing the other hand on the athlete's sacrum, gently tractioning the sacrum upward and rotating the hips toward the floor to open the low back.

5. For PNF, the athlete attempts to roll the hips down to the table against the resistance of the assister's hands.

6. For the stretch, the assister increases the athlete's hip and low back rotation with traction of the sacrum away from the center of the back and then rotates the hip and low back toward the floor. The athlete should keep the upper body relaxed, with both shoulders remaining on the table.

7. Repeat the PNF series two or more times and explore the different angles of the stretch.

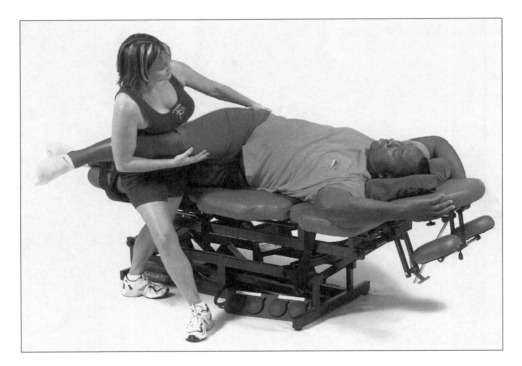

GLUTES AND DEEP ROTATORS

1. The athlete lies on his or her back, bringing the leg at a 90-degree angle across the body, parallel with the floor.
2. The assister places a hand on the side of the athlete's knee to externally rotate the femur and bring the foot toward the opposite shoulder. The assister places the athlete's leg on the assister's shoulder, grasping the table for leverage.
3. For PNF, the assister moves the hand to the back side of the athlete's knee while the athlete gently pushes into the hand.
4. The assister tractions the athlete's hip gently up and out of its socket using the table and the assister's body for leverage.
5. The closer the athlete's leg is toward his or her chest, the deeper the stretch in gluteus maximus. The more the leg externally rotates, the deeper the stretch in the rotators.
6. Repeat two or more times and explore different angles of the stretch.

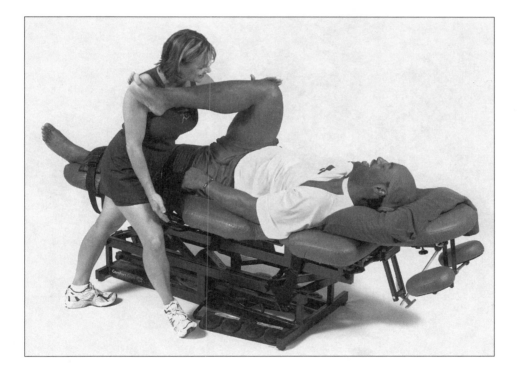

GLUTEUS MEDIUS

1. The assister brings the athlete's knee to the center of the chest and the athlete's foot down toward the opposite hip. The photo shows how the assister uses his or her body for leverage.

2. For PNF, the athlete presses the knee into the assister's hand.

3. The assister tractions the athlete's hip gently upward by lifting the hip of the leg being stretched slightly off the floor to create more space in the hip joint before increasing the hip flexion and adduction to stretch.

4. If the athlete feels a pinching in the front of the hip, the assister should apply more force on the foot.

5. Repeat two or more times and explore different angles of the stretch.

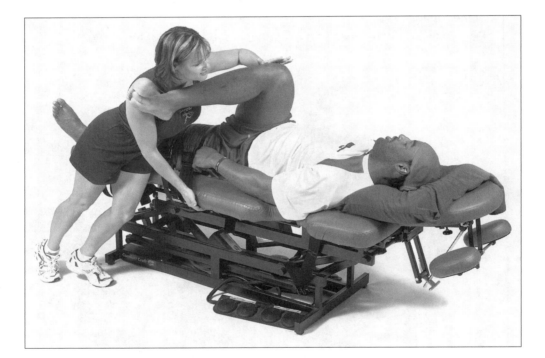

HAMSTRINGS

1. The assister straightens the athlete's leg out into hip flexion, keeping the knee as straight as possible and opening the leg slightly to the side.
2. The assister places one hand on the athlete's heel to traction the leg up and out of the hip socket and places the other hand on the back of the hamstrings.
3. For PNF, the athlete pushes with the entire leg into the assister's hands.
4. For the stretch, the assister tractions the leg upward and out of the socket and gently increases hip flexion.
5. Repeat two or more times and explore different angles of the stretch.

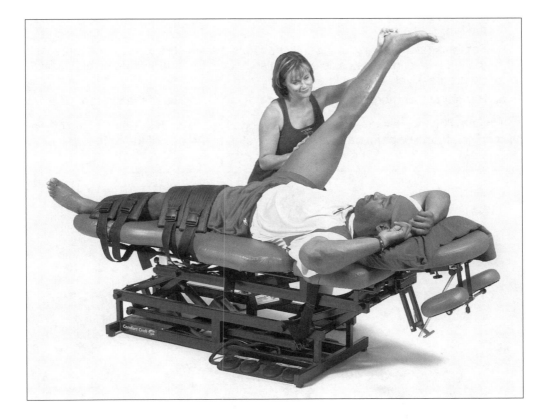

HIP FLEXORS

1. Restraints aren't used for this stretch. The athlete lies on his or her side and drops the bottom leg forward off the edge of the table with a bent knee. The athlete extends the other leg backward and grasps the top of the table with the top arm.

2. The assister extends the athlete's top leg backward with the knee flexed slightly and places the athlete's shin across the front of the assister with the athlete's foot against the assister's hip.

3. The assister places one hand above the athlete's knee and the other hand under the foot with the assister's fingers on the athlete's heel.

4. For PNF, the athlete pulls his or her top knee toward the other leg by flexing at the hip.

5. For the stretch, the assister gently tractions the athlete's leg out and increases the hip extension. The assister can also stretch the quadriceps in this position by progressively adding knee flexion.

6. Repeat two or more times and explore different angles of the stretch.

If the hip flexors are extremely tight, it is a good idea to do this stretch at the beginning of the routine or before the lateral line stretch at the end of the routine.

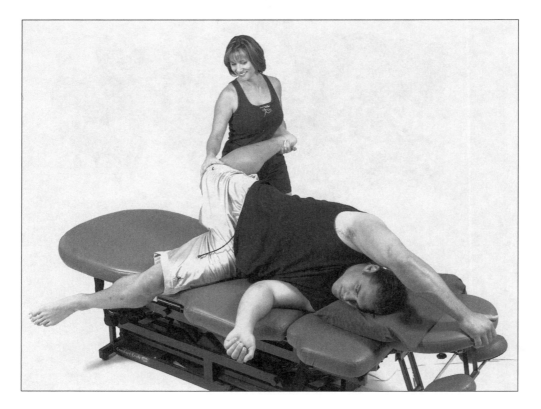

LATERAL LINE

1. The athlete rolls onto his or her back, and the assister takes both of the athlete's legs over to the side and drops the leg being stretched under top leg. The assister provides support for the athlete's legs by placing his or her own legs underneath them and by placing both hands on them from above.
2. The athlete reaches upward with the same arm and hand as the leg being stretched.
3. For PNF, the athlete pushes against the assister with the bottom leg.
4. For the stretch, the assister increases traction and lateral flexion of the bottom leg. The more the assister drops the athlete's legs toward the floor, the deeper the stretch.
5. To increase the stretch, on an exhalation the athletes roll the gluteal muscles back down to the table as the assister increases the lateral flexion and traction of both legs.
6. Repeat two or more times and explore different angles of the stretch.

We recommend beginning and ending the lower body routine with this stretch. You can stretch both sides and check to see if the athlete's body is more flexible at the end of the routine.

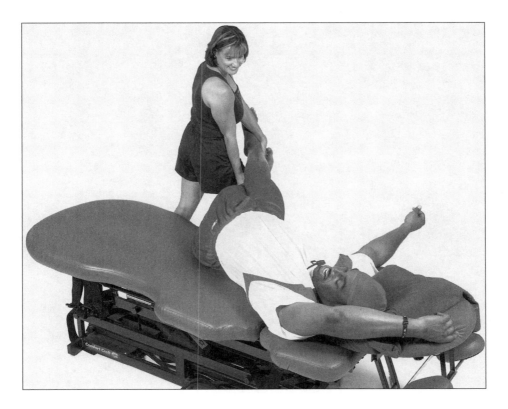

We have offered here just a sample of the assisted stretches we do in our clinic and teach at our institute. We hope the information presented in this book will encourage you to implement or continue your own flexibility program using some of the principles and methods of our Stretch to Win system. Our goal is for you to realize your true performance potential and avoid injury by maximizing your flexibility.

glossary

Types of Flexibility

Active flexibility is the measure of the range of motion (ROM) in the presence of active muscle contraction.

Ballistic flexibility refers to the ability to use ROM with explosive speed, thereby facilitating the stretch reflex.

Dynamic flexibility refers to the ability to use ROM to execute physical activity at either normal or rapid speed.

Functional flexibility refers to the ability to apply sufficient dynamic and ballistic flexibility to perform any movement necessary for a specific activity or sport; proper muscular strength is a crucial component.

Passive flexibility is the measure of ROM in the absence of active muscle contraction.

Relative flexibility relates to the tendency of the body to take the path of least resistance during functional movement patterns. This type of flexibility can result in dysfunction and pain.

Static flexibility relates to ROM about a joint with no emphasis on speed; it is controlled passive movement taken to the point of resistance.

Types of Stretching

Active-assisted stretching is initiated by the person being stretched, performing an active contraction of the agonist muscle group until that movement is restricted by the tight antagonist group. At this point, the person relaxes the agonist and then the partner assists by striving for further movement in the same direction to increase the flexibility of the antagonist.

Example: After performing the straight leg raise until restricted by the tight hamstring muscles, the athlete relaxes while his or her partner takes the leg further up into the range. This would include reciprocal inhibition by starting with active range of motion (AROM), then passive range of motion (PROM) by outside force.

Active stretching (AROM of varying intensities, durations, and frequencies) is accomplished when the person who is stretching uses his or her own muscles to move through the range of motion without using any external force. The person may perform active stretching statically, dynamically, or ballistically.

*Indicates terms specific to the Stretch to Win system.

*Assisted stretching** as done in the Stretch to Win (STW) system is a modified proprioceptive neuromuscular facilitation (PNF) technique. STW assisted stretching is performed by a certified flexibility specialist with the client on a treatment table or on the floor or field. When assisted stretching takes place on a treatment table, comfortable straps are used to stabilize the limb or part of the body that is not being worked on, thus facilitating complete relaxation of the person being stretched and enhancing the effectiveness of the actions of the specialist. In contrast to traditional PNF, clients using the STW system contract their muscles 25 to 50 percent (versus 100 percent) and hold until they feel the release, approximately 3 to 4 seconds (versus 6 to 10 seconds), for a more effective relaxation response. See also *proprioceptive neuromuscular facilitation.*

Ballistic stretching involves bouncing, rebounding, bobbing, and kicking movements that are usually rhythmic in nature. Although its use is controversial, ballistic stretching is considered a necessary part of sport-specific training when used within the context of a total flexibility program rather than as a solitary technique.

Example: dancers, gymnasts, and martial artists will repetitively kick, bounce, and flip their bodies in multiple ways and directions only after first raising their core body temperature by means of a good warm-up.

Contract-relax (hold-relax) technique is a proprioceptive neuromuscular facilitation (PNF) technique that begins with the target muscle group in a mildly lengthened position. The muscles then perform a moderate isometric contraction for 6 to 15 seconds against practitioner resistance. The muscle is allowed a few seconds of relaxation, and then the practitioner slowly deepens the stretch with passive movement. This procedure can be repeated several times as comfort and tissue response allows. See also *proprioceptive neuromuscular facilitation.*

Contract-relax-agonist-contract (CRAC) technique is a proprioceptive neuromuscular facilitation (PNF) technique that is very similar to the contract-relax technique except that after the relaxation phase, the agonist (muscle opposing the one being stretched) is actively contracted by the athlete until he or she feels the movement being stopped by the sensation of stretch in the antagonist. At this point, the athlete relaxes in the new stretch position and starts the sequence all over again several times as comfort and tissue response allows. See also *contract-relax technique* and *proprioceptive neuromuscular facilitation.*

*Core four stretches** affect the low back, pelvis, and hip area, commonly called the core of the body. The core four include stretches for the hip flexors, the gluteus complex, the quadratus lumborum, and the latissimus dorsi.

Dynamic stretching involves progressive amplitudes and arcs of movement performed in a swinging or pendulum manner and is often confused with ballistic stretching. It is a more activity- or sport-specific form of stretching and can be done as part of a warm-up.

Example: Competitive swimmers sometimes perform large swinging movements of their arms immediately before jumping off the race block, and baseball players may swing the bat around in different directions before coming to the plate.

Passive-active stretching is slightly different from passive stretching in that the stretch is initially accomplished by an outside force, then the person being stretched attempts to hold the stretch by isometrically contracting the agonist muscle. This is done in order to strengthen the weak agonist that is being reflexively inhibited by the tight antagonist muscle.

Example: The athlete lies on the back as the partner performs a straight leg raise. When the athlete feels the stretch, the partner lets go while the athlete activates the quadriceps to hold the position.

Passive stretching (PROM) occurs when the person being stretched does not contribute to the range of motion. This form of stretching usually involves an outside agent such as a partner, towel, or other apparatus that applies the force.

Example: The athlete lies on the back and the partner performs a straight leg raise until the athlete feels a stretch, at which time the partner holds the position.

Proprioceptive neuromuscular facilitation (PNF) is defined by Dorothy Voss, PT, as "methods of promoting or hastening the response of the neuromuscular mechanism through stimulation of the proprioceptors." Originated and developed by Herman Kabat, MD, PhD, and Margaret Knott, PT, in the 1940s to treat patients with paralysis, it was modified in the 1970s by physical therapists and athletic trainers to increase and maintain flexibility and range of motion in healthy people. PNF stretching techniques may also be known as modified PNF, NF, or scientific stretching for sport (3-S technique). There are multiple PNF techniques: see *contract-relax technique* and *contract-relax-agonist-contract.*

Self-myofascial release (sMFR) is a highly effective method that uses a ball, foam roller, or other tool to help reduce or eliminate soft tissue restrictions, trigger points, adhesions, and tight spots that inhibit both strength and flexibility. This technique is especially beneficial when used before stretching to warm-up the tissue and release specific areas.

Static stretching is the most simple and commonly used type of stretching; it involves a person placing a muscle or group of muscles in a lengthened position and then maintaining that position for a variable period of time ranging from a few seconds to several minutes. By holding the position for a sustained period without movement, the stretch reflex can be bypassed.

Example: The athlete lies on the back and performs a straight leg raise, holding it at the position of stretch.

*****Stretch wave** is a metaphor used to help people visualize a stretch as being made up of undulations of movement coordinated with proper breathing. This metaphor comes from observing that many physiological and kinesiological processes in the body occur in waves, from the light waves that stimulate the retina in vision to the pulsing waves of the blood in arteries and veins. See also *undulating stretching.*

*****Stretching matrix** is the name we use for our method of developing a stretching program. It begins with the core four stretches for the low back, pelvis, and hips, and builds outward to the rest of the trunk and extremities. The program progresses in a logical and comprehensive fashion, stretching regions of muscle and fascia that are both short and long as well as both deep and superficial. See also, *core four stretches.*

*****Traction** is the physical act of decompressing the two surfaces of a joint. Manually decompressing the joint surfaces triggers a stretch in the joint capsule. This response within the joint capsule causes reflexive relaxation of the muscles that share the same innervation source and cross on or near the joint.

*Undulating stretching is the term we use to describe the difference between the Stretch To Win technique and traditional techniques of stretching. Instead of holding a stretch, athletes undulate the stretch, oscillating at various tempos and directions as their tissue dictates.

Anatomical and Physiological Terms

*Anatomy Trains is the term for a system of myofascial meridians (also called myofascial lines) as discovered and defined by advanced Rolfer and creator of Kinesis Myofascial Integration Thomas Myers. In the simplest terms, the system shows how muscles are strung together longitudinally to form a supporting tensile network for the skeleton.

Autonomic nervous system (ANS) is the part of the nervous system that is not typically consciously controlled. It is commonly divided into two usually antagonistic subsystems: the sympathetic and parasympathetic nervous systems. The autonomic nervous system controls such vital functions as heart rate and breathing, and originates in the central nervous system (brain and spinal cord). See also, *sympathetic nervous system* and *parasympathetic nervous system*.

Collagen is the second most prevalent structural material in the human body after water. Connective tissue, or fascia, is primarily made of collagen, elastin, and water. Collagen's main structural property is its great tensile strength; therefore, tissues that contain more collagen than elastin, such as tendons, are resistant to pulling forces.

Connective tissue is any type of biological tissue with an extensive extracellular matrix. It often serves to support, bind together, and protect the tissue. There are four basic types of connective tissue—bone, blood, cartilage, and connective tissue proper. Connective tissue proper includes dense connective tissue such as ligaments and tendons, loose connective tissue that helps hold organs in place, reticular connective tissue that forms a soft skeleton to support the lymphoid organs, and adipose or fat tissue.

Elastin is a protein in connective tissue that is elastic and allows many tissues in the body to resume their shape after stretching or contracting.

Extracelluar matrix is any material that is part of a tissue but not part of any cell. It is the defining feature of connective tissue.

Fascia refers to the specialized connective tissue layer which surrounds muscles, bones, and joints, providing support and protection and giving structure to the body. It consists of three layers: the *superficial fascia*, the *deep fascia*, and the *subserous fascia*. The particular fascia that surrounds the muscles is called myofascia. See also, *myofascia*.

Joint capsule is the connective tissue structure that encapsulates joints and plays an essential role in optimizing joint function both nutritionally and mechanically. The capsule has a fibrous outer layer that serves to enclose the joint structure and restrict its range of motion. The inner layer secretes synovial fluid, which lubricates and provides nutrients to the joint.

Myofascia is the name of specialized connective tissue that surrounds each muscle and tendon, and merges with the fascia of the bone.

Parasympathetic nervous system (PNS) is one of two divisions of the autonomic nervous system. Sometimes called the *rest and digest* system, the PNS conserves energy as it slows the heart rate, increases intestinal and glandular activity, and relaxes the gastrointestinal tract. Traditionally it is said that the PNS acts in a reciprocal manner to the effects of the sympathetic nervous system. However, because some tissues are innervated by both systems, the effects are also synergistic. The cells of the PNS are located in the brain stem (cranium) and the sacral part of the central nervous system. See also *autonomic nervous system* and *sympathetic nervous system*.

*__Rebound effect__ refers to the tendency of muscle that has just been stretched to tighten up again immediately afterward. This may happen from stretching with too much intensity or for too great a duration or may be an indication of a high level of waste products or toxic matter in the body.

__Sympathetic nervous system__ (SNS): is part of the autonomic nervous system, which also includes the parasympathetic nervous system. The SNS activates what is often termed the *fight or flight response*. Sympathetic nerves originate inside the vertebral column, toward the middle of the spinal cord, beginning at the first thoracic segment of the spinal cord and extending into the second or third lumbar segments. See also *autonomic nervous system* and *parasympathetic nervous system*.

__Stretch reflex__ occurs when a muscle is stretched such that the primary sensory fibers of the muscle spindle, located in the muscle belly, respond to both the velocity and the degree of stretch, and send this information to the spinal cord. Likewise, secondary sensory fibers detect and send information about the degree of stretch (but not the velocity) to the central nervous system. The conveyance of this information to the motor nerves activates the extrafusal fibers of the muscle, causing them to contract, thereby reducing or even stopping the stretch.

references

Alter, Michael. 2004. *Science of flexibility*, 3rd ed. Champaign, IL: Human Kinetics.

Cook, Gray. 2003. *Athletic body in balance*. Champaign, IL: Human Kinetics.

Frederick, Ann. 1997. Proprioceptive neuromuscular facilitation: Effectiveness in increasing functional range of motion in dancers and other athletes. Unpublished thesis.

Johns, R.J., and V. Wright. 1962. Relative importance of various tissues in joint stiffness. *Journal of Applied Physiology*, 17(5), 824-828.

Kendall, Florence P, and Elizabeth Kendall McCreary. 1993. *Muscles: Testing and Function*. Philadelphia: Lippincott, Williams and Wilkins.

Mühlemann and Cimino. 1990. Therapeutic muscle stretching. In W.I. Hammer (Ed.), *Functional soft tissue examination and treatment by manual methods*. The extremities (pp. 251-275). Gaithersburg, MD: Aspen.

Myers, Thomas W. 2001. *Anatomy trains*. London: Churchill Livingstone.

National Strength and Conditioning Association (NSCA). 2000. *Essentials of strength and conditioning*. Thomas Baechle and Roger Earle (eds). Champaign: IL Human Kinetics.

Oschman, James L. 2003. *Energy medicine in therapeutics and human performance*. London Butterworth-Heinemann.

Rhea, Matthew R., Stephen D. Ball, Wayne T. Phillips, and Lee N. Burkett. 2002. A comparison of linear and daily undulating periodized programs with equated volume and intensity for strength. *Journal of Strength Conditioning Research* May 16(2):250-255.

Siff, Mel C. 2003. *Supertraining*, 6th ed. Denver, CO: Supertraining Institute.

For an updated listing of stretching resources, visit our products page at www.stretchtowin.com.

index

Note: The italicized *f* and *t* following page numbers refer to figures and tables, respectively.

about the authors

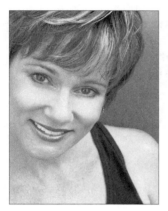

Ann Frederick is the director of flexibility training for the Stretch to Win Clinic, where she has worked with many elite athletes, including Philadelphia Eagles star quarterback Donovan McNabb and numerous Olympians and members of the NFL, MLB, and NHL. Ann was the first flexibility specialist ever to work at the Olympics, consulting with the 1996 U.S. wrestling team and both the 2000 and 2004 U.S. track teams.

For more than 35 years, Ann has studied, performed, and taught movement through multiple dance disciplines. In 1997, upon completion of her studies, Frederick defended her master's thesis and established that her stretching technique outperformed conventional methods with lasting flexibility gains of 36 to 52 percent. She continually refined and improved these techniques, which ultimately developed into the Stretch to Win system of flexibility training and stretching. Today, professional athletes and Olympians from all over the world use this system to achieve higher levels of performance.

Ann is a member of the International Association of Structural Integrators and is part of the associate faculty at Arizona State University.

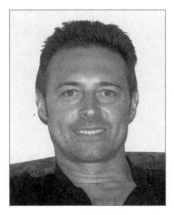

Chris Frederick is the director of sports and orthopedic rehabilitation at the Stretch to Win Clinic. After an injury sidelined his professional dance career, Chris went on to receive his degree in manual orthopedic physical therapy from Hunter College, City University of New York. To get a well-rounded background in many disciplines, Chris trained privately with several master physical therapists, rolfers, chiropractors, osteopaths, two chi kung and tai chi masters, and an Olympic strength coach.

As a result of his education and training, Chris lends a nontraditional, complementary approach to flexibility training, physical therapy, sport rehabilitation, and fitness. Using the Stretch To Win system of flexibility training and stretching, he has designed many effective injury-prevention programs for both professional and collegiate athletes and sport teams as well as professional dancers and dance companies. Chris is a member of the American Physical Therapy Association, the International Association of Structural Integrators, and the International Association of Dance, Medicine and Science.

The Fredericks are also renowned international speakers and codirectors of the International Institute of Flexibility Sciences located in Tempe, Arizona. There, they train and certify professionals to become flexibility specialists who may use the Stretch To Win system to enhance their current careers. The Fredericks are dedicated to advancing the emerging field of flexibility sciences by promoting and engaging in research on connective tissue and related topics.

The Fredericks reside in Tempe, Arizona.

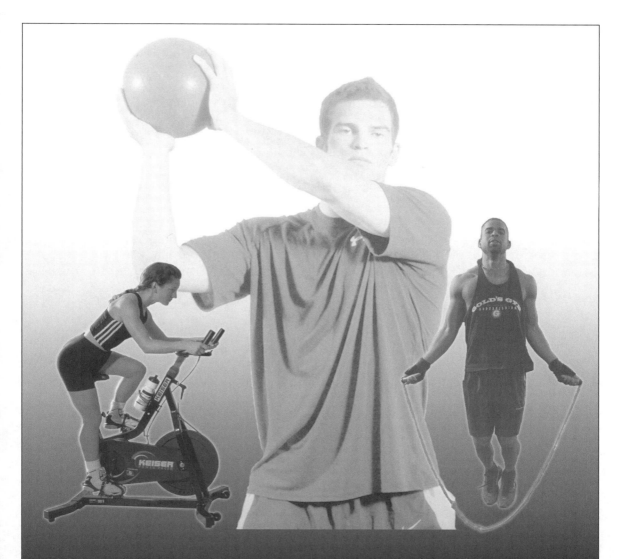
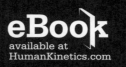